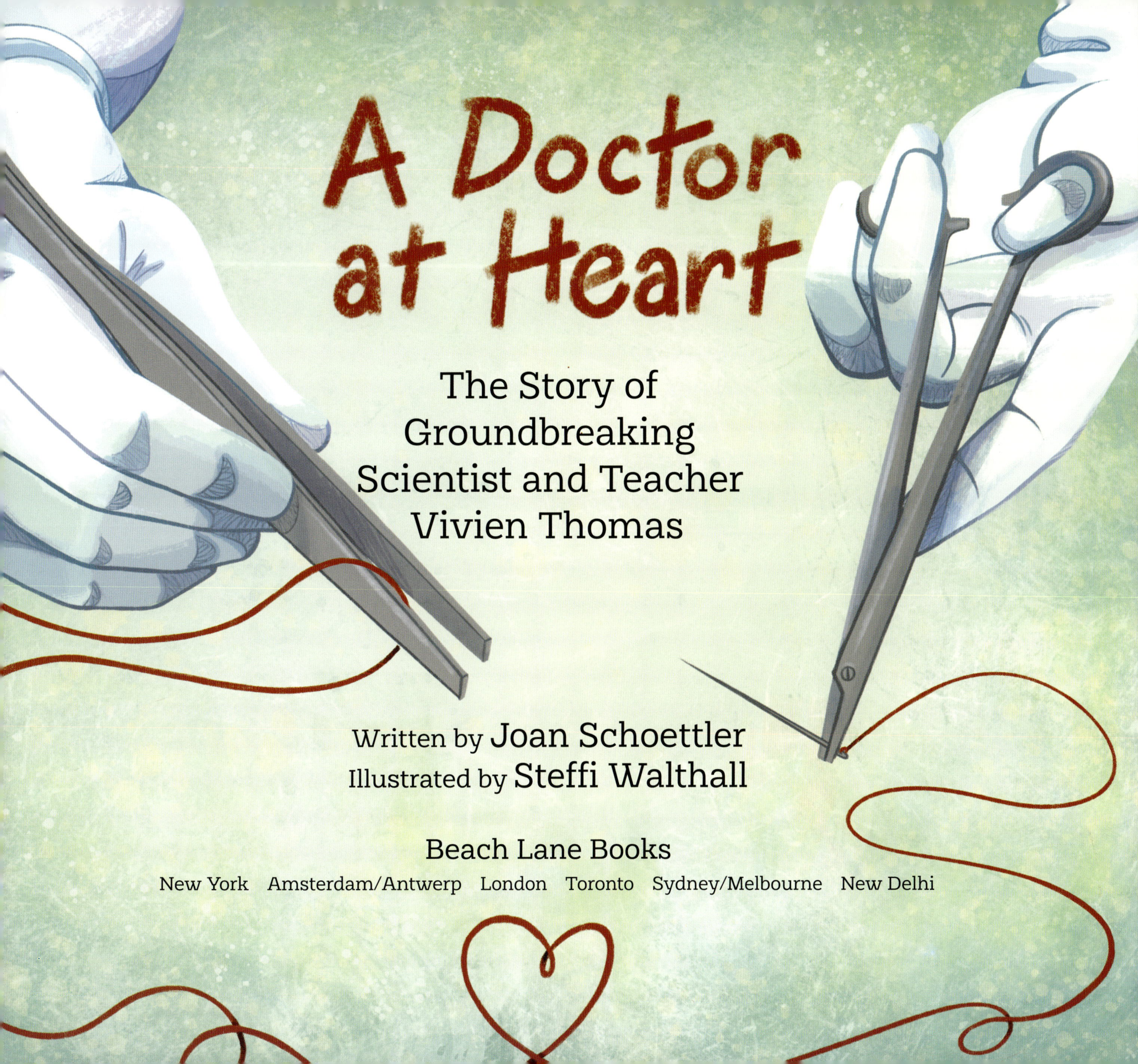

A Doctor at Heart

The Story of Groundbreaking Scientist and Teacher Vivien Thomas

Written by Joan Schoettler
Illustrated by Steffi Walthall

Beach Lane Books
New York Amsterdam/Antwerp London Toronto Sydney/Melbourne New Delhi

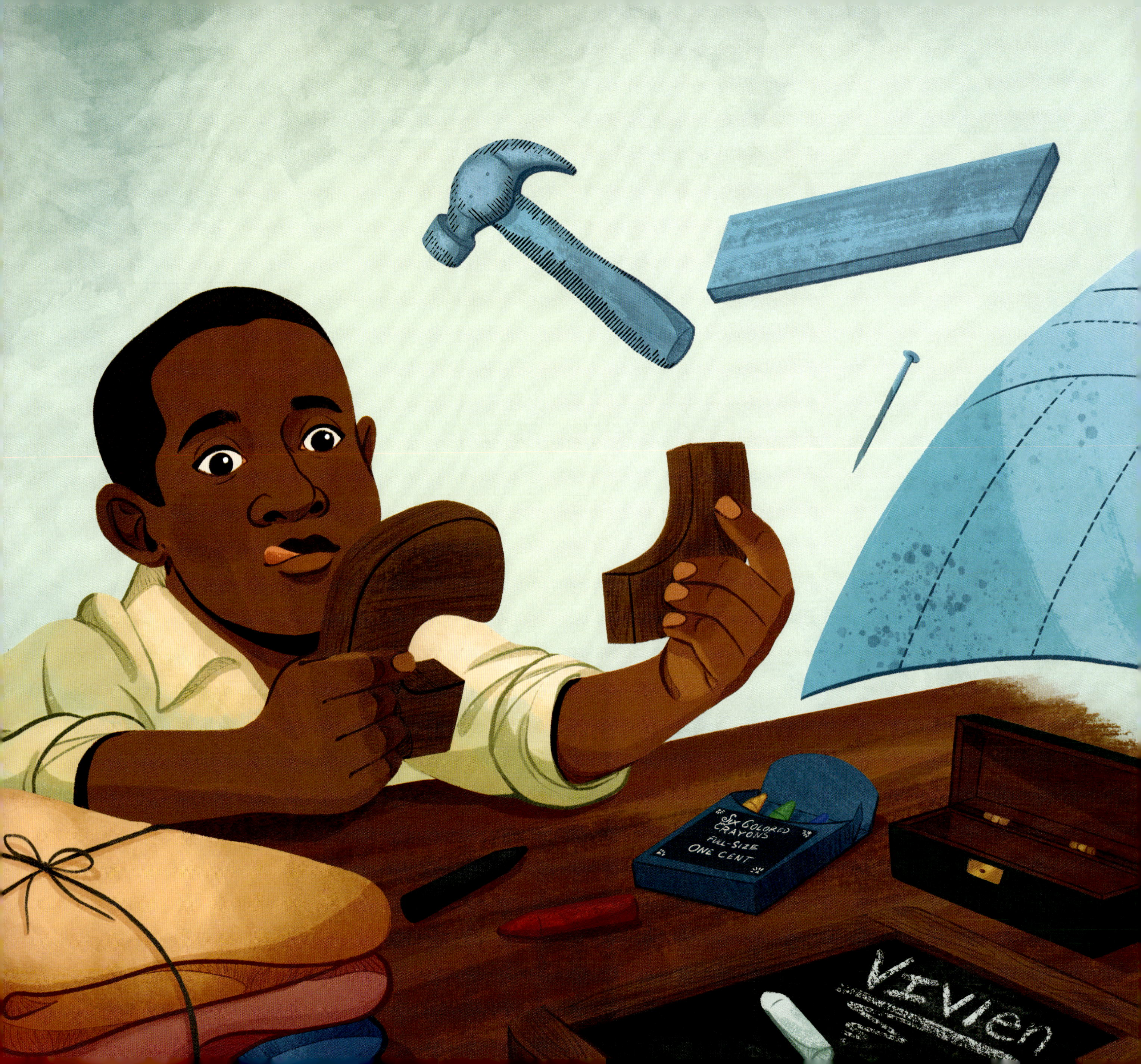
Six Colored
Crayons
Full-Size
One Cent
Vivien

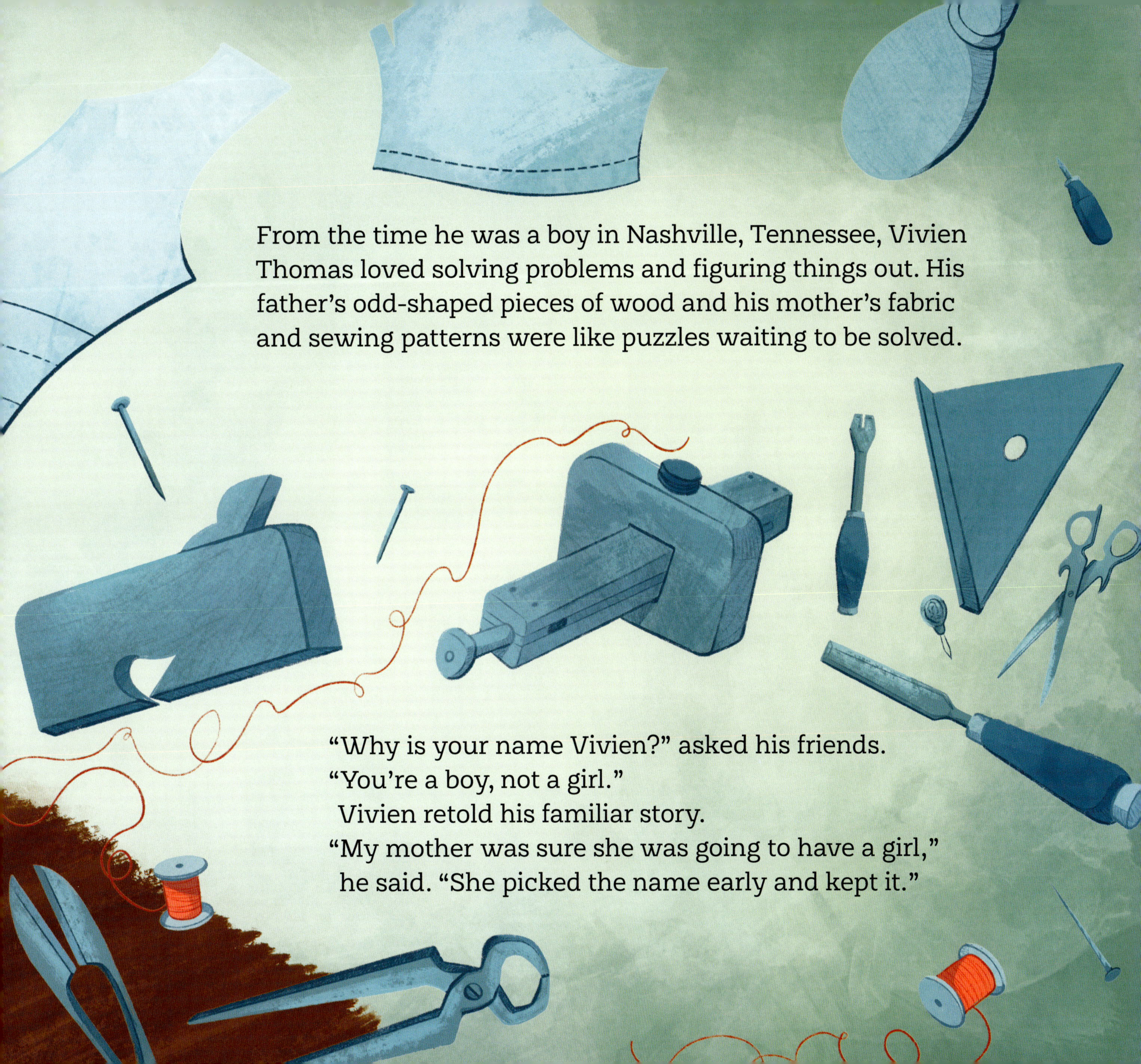

From the time he was a boy in Nashville, Tennessee, Vivien Thomas loved solving problems and figuring things out. His father's odd-shaped pieces of wood and his mother's fabric and sewing patterns were like puzzles waiting to be solved.

"Why is your name Vivien?" asked his friends. "You're a boy, not a girl."

Vivien retold his familiar story.

"My mother was sure she was going to have a girl," he said. "She picked the name early and kept it."

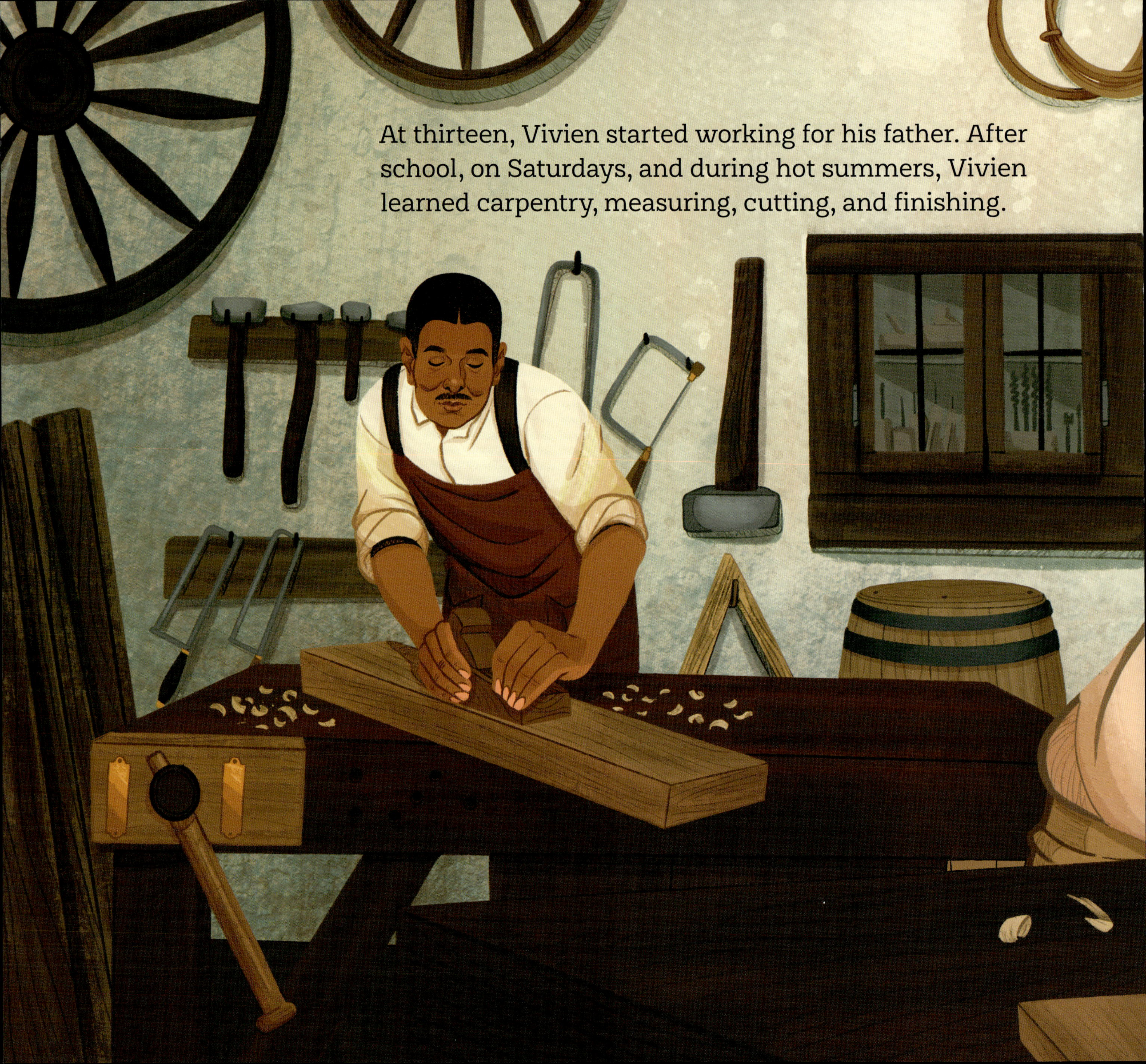

At thirteen, Vivien started working for his father. After school, on Saturdays, and during hot summers, Vivien learned carpentry, measuring, cutting, and finishing.

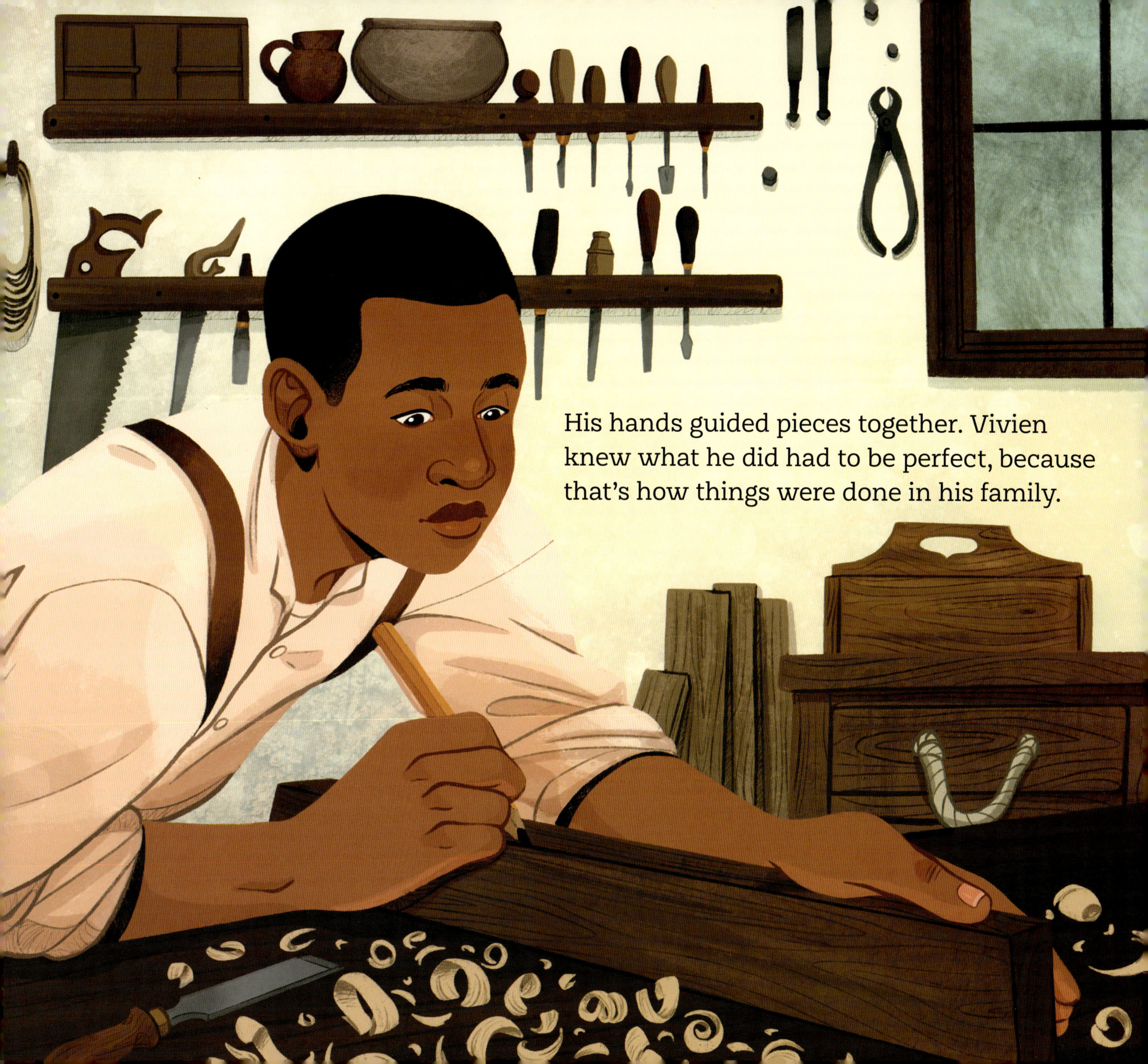

His hands guided pieces together. Vivien knew what he did had to be perfect, because that's how things were done in his family.

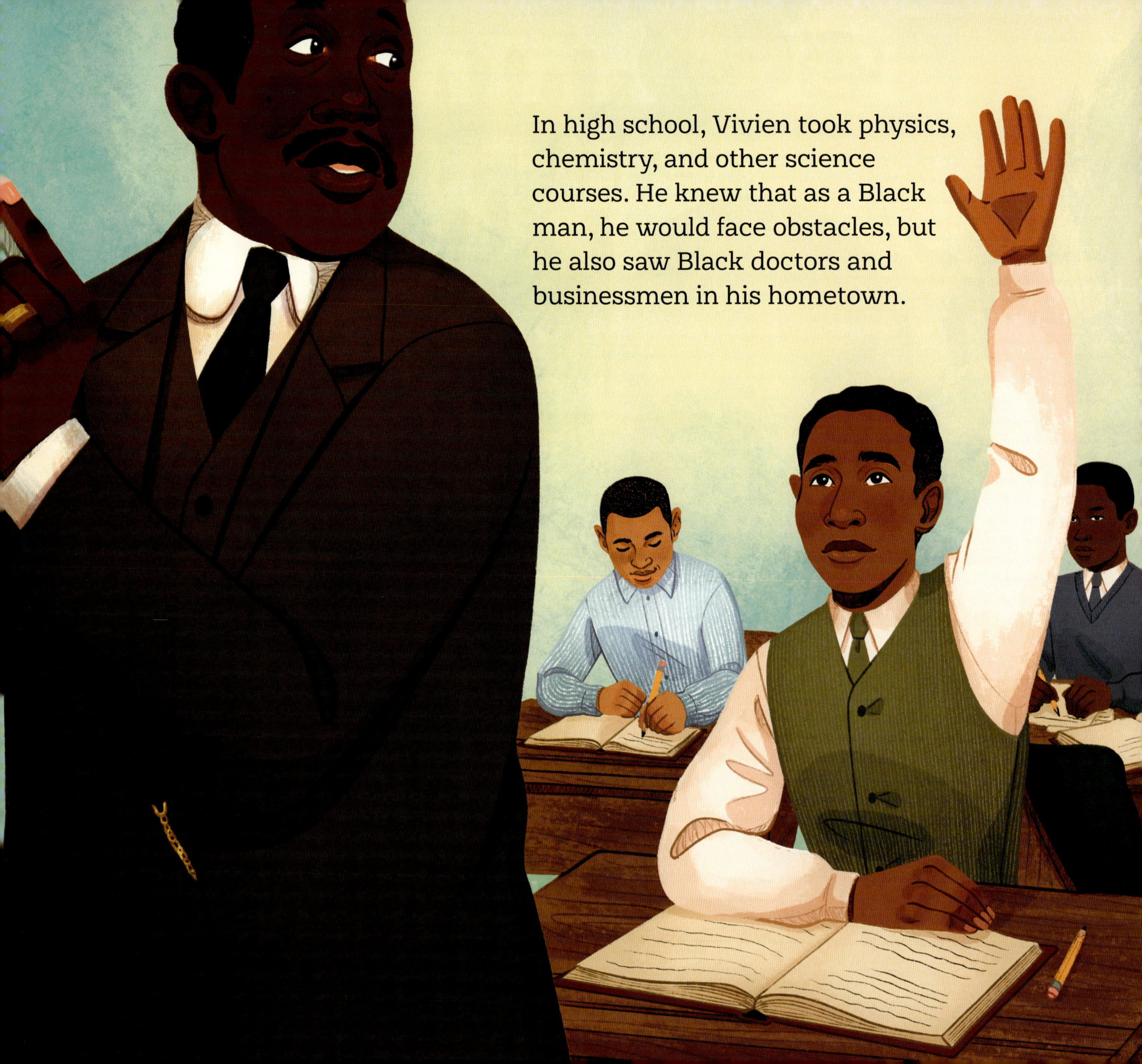

In high school, Vivien took physics, chemistry, and other science courses. He knew that as a Black man, he would face obstacles, but he also saw Black doctors and businessmen in his hometown.

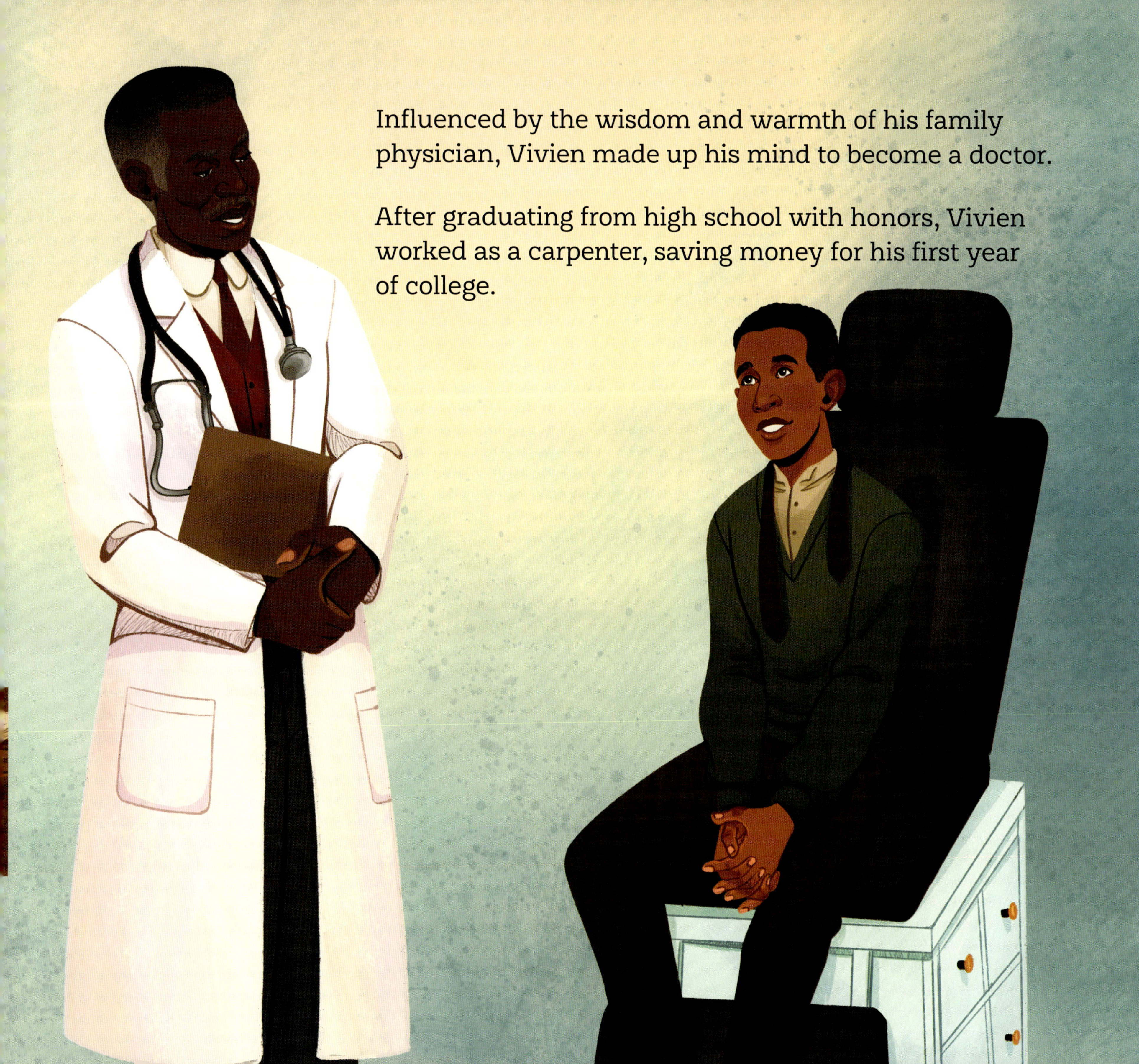

Influenced by the wisdom and warmth of his family physician, Vivien made up his mind to become a doctor.

After graduating from high school with honors, Vivien worked as a carpenter, saving money for his first year of college.

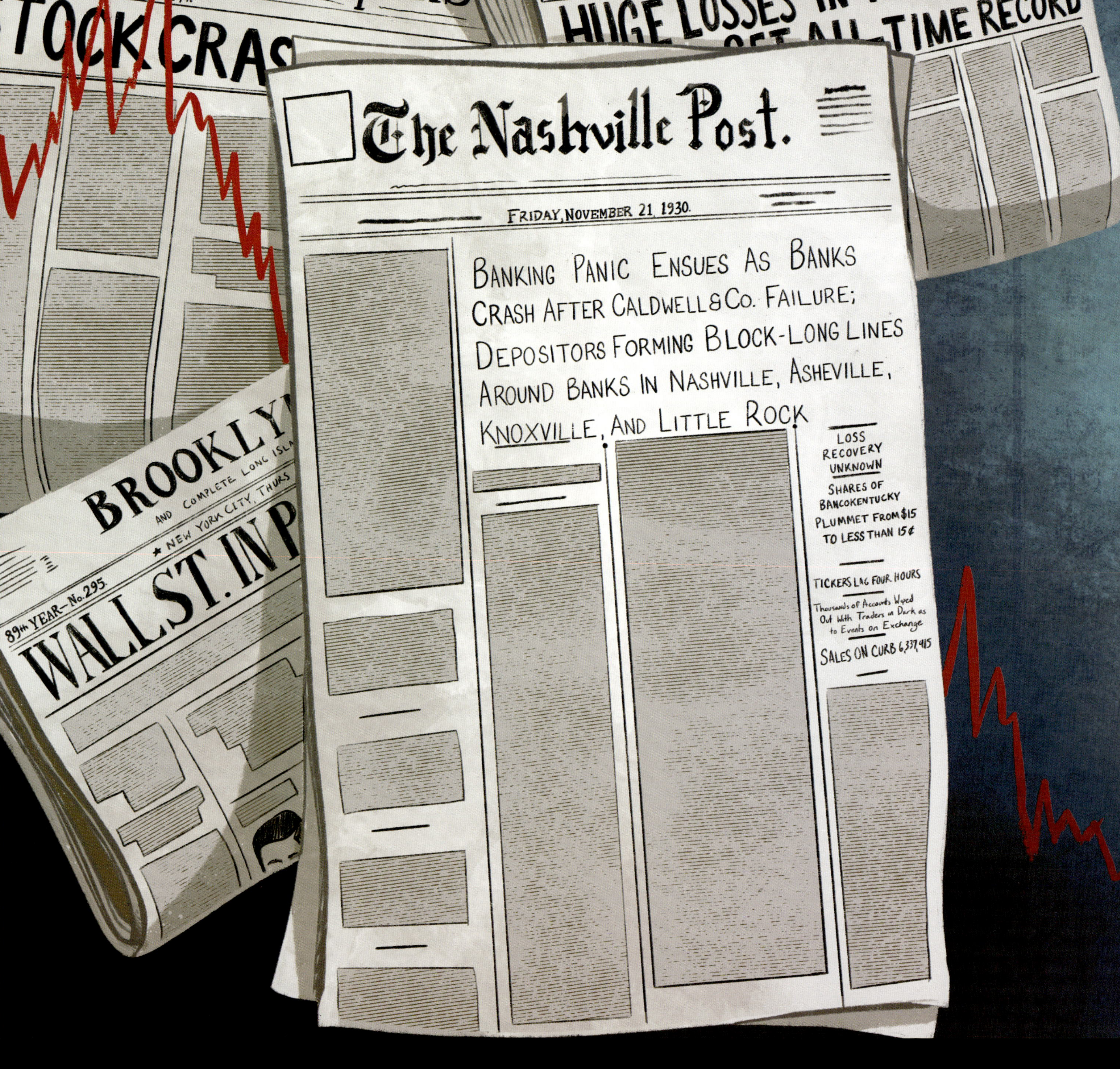
STOCK CRAS
HUGE LOSSES IN
TIME RECORD
The Nashville Post.
FRIDAY, NOVEMBER 21 1930.
BANKING PANIC ENSUES AS BANKS CRASH AFTER CALDWELL & CO. FAILURE; DEPOSITORS FORMING BLOCK-LONG LINES AROUND BANKS IN NASHVILLE, ASHEVILLE, KNOXVILLE, AND LITTLE ROCK
LOSS RECOVERY UNKNOWN
SHARES OF BANCOKENTUCKY PLUMMET FROM $15 TO LESS THAN 15¢
TICKERS LAG FOUR HOURS
Thousands of Accounts Wiped Out With Traders in Dark as to Events on Exchange
SALES ON CURB 6,337,415
BROOKLY
AND COMPLETE LONG ISL
NEW YORK CITY, THURS
89th YEAR— No. 295.
WALL ST. IN P

Vivien was gaining valuable skills and earning money. But then, in November 1930, a financial disaster struck. Vivien's bank failed, and his entire college savings were lost. "I was dumbfounded, discouraged, angry, depressed, you name it," said Vivien. Yet his desire to become a doctor held fast.

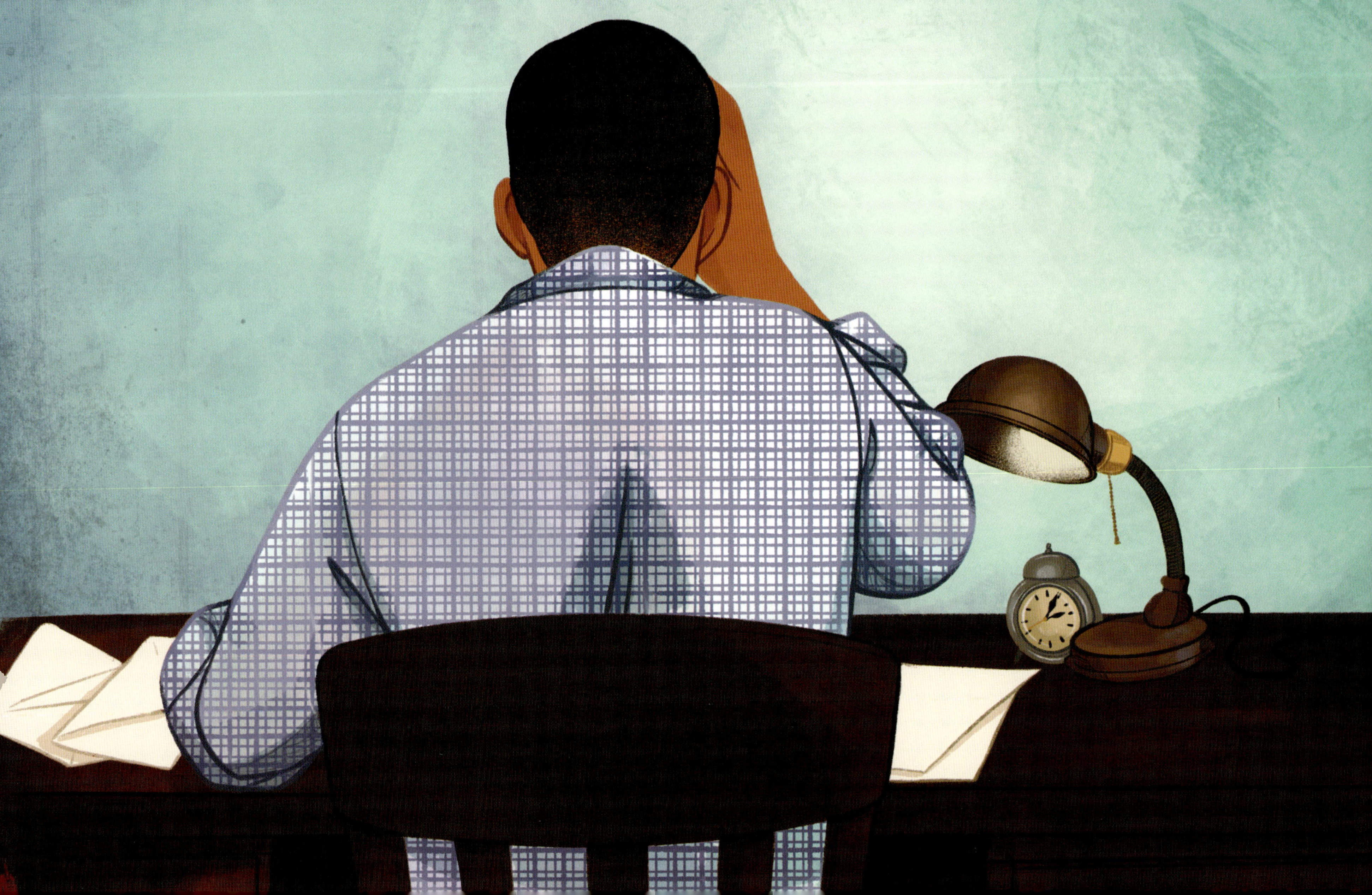

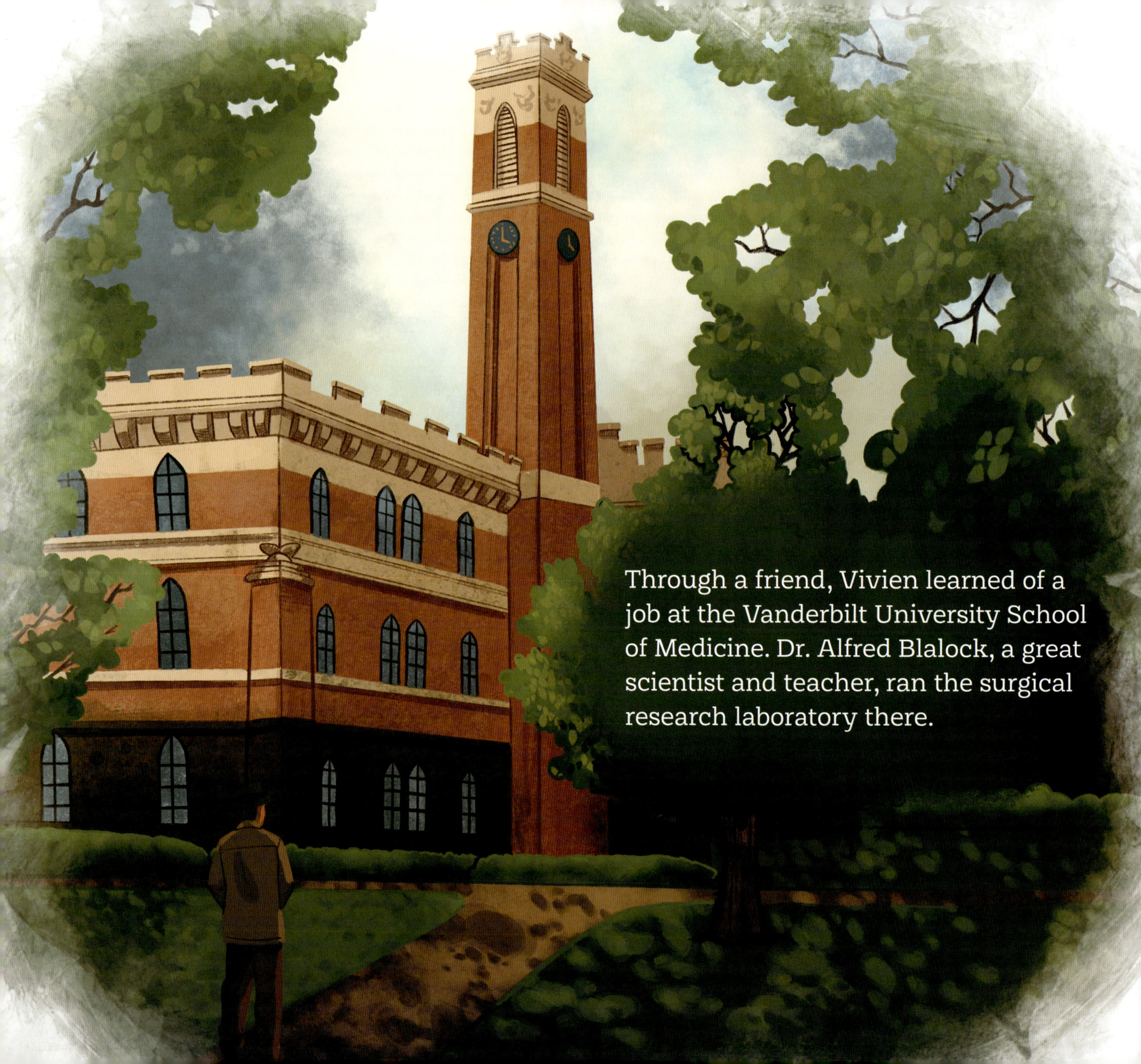

Through a friend, Vivien learned of a job at the Vanderbilt University School of Medicine. Dr. Alfred Blalock, a great scientist and teacher, ran the surgical research laboratory there.

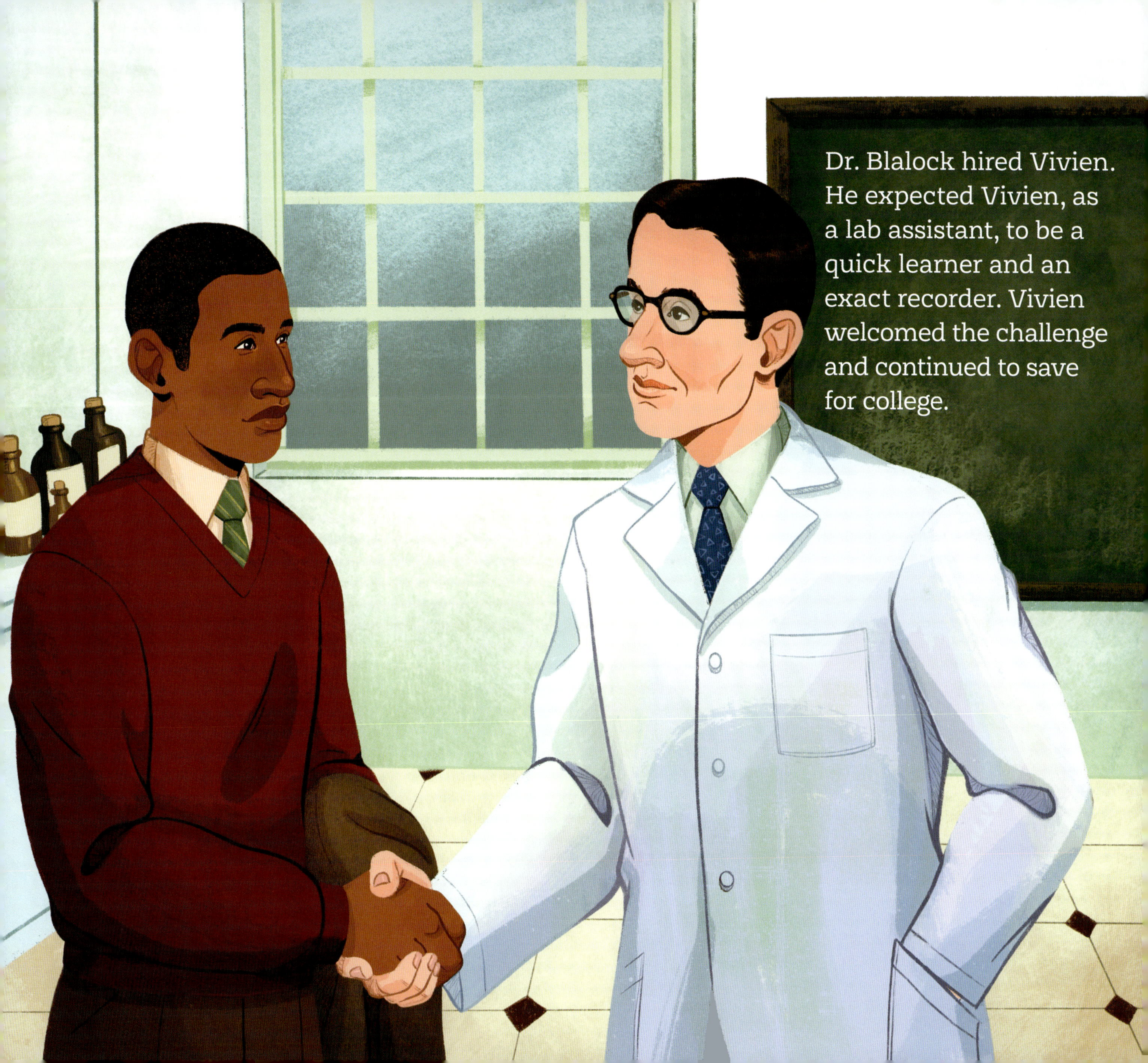

Dr. Blalock hired Vivien. He expected Vivien, as a lab assistant, to be a quick learner and an exact recorder. Vivien welcomed the challenge and continued to save for college.

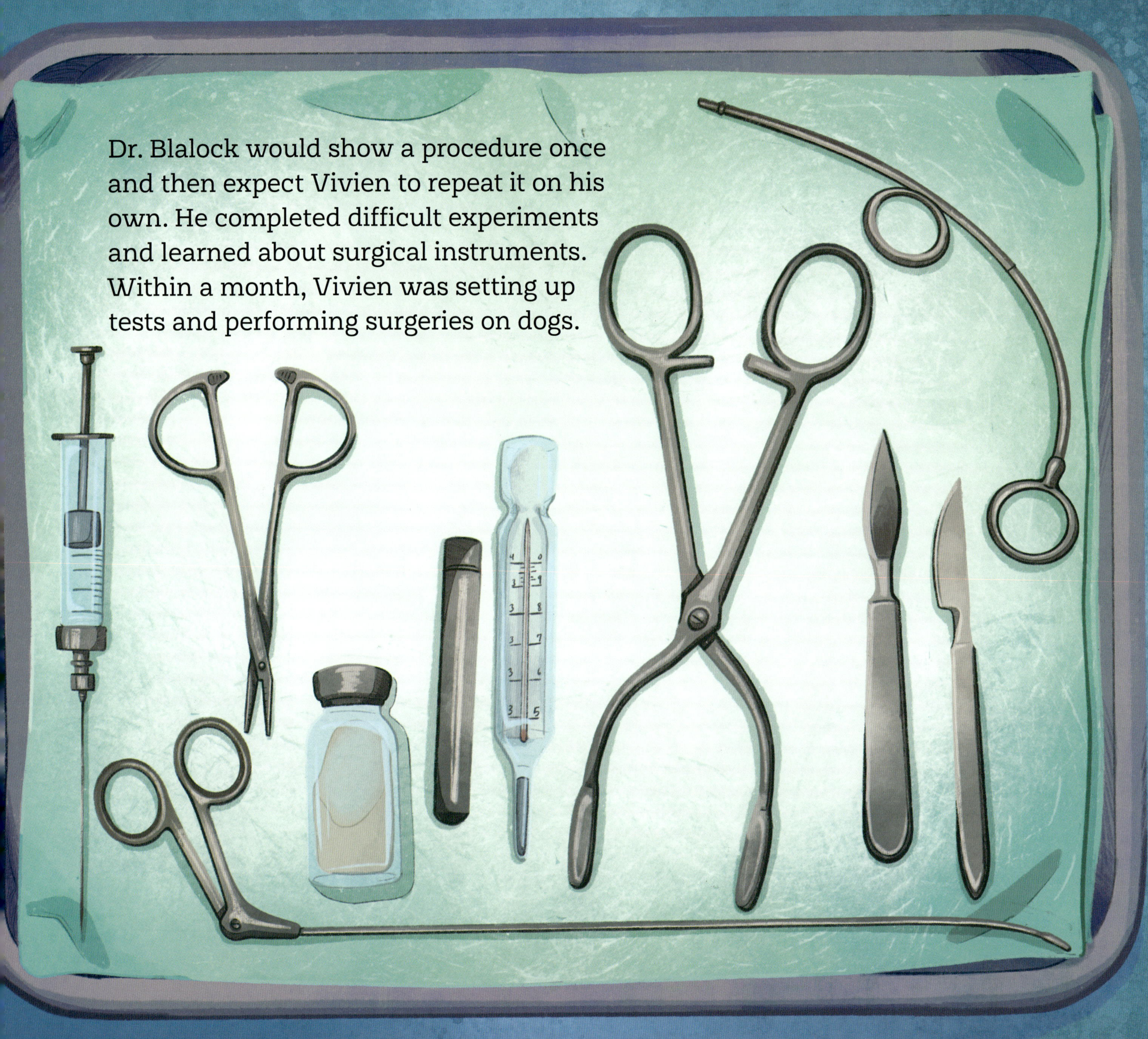

Dr. Blalock would show a procedure once and then expect Vivien to repeat it on his own. He completed difficult experiments and learned about surgical instruments. Within a month, Vivien was setting up tests and performing surgeries on dogs.

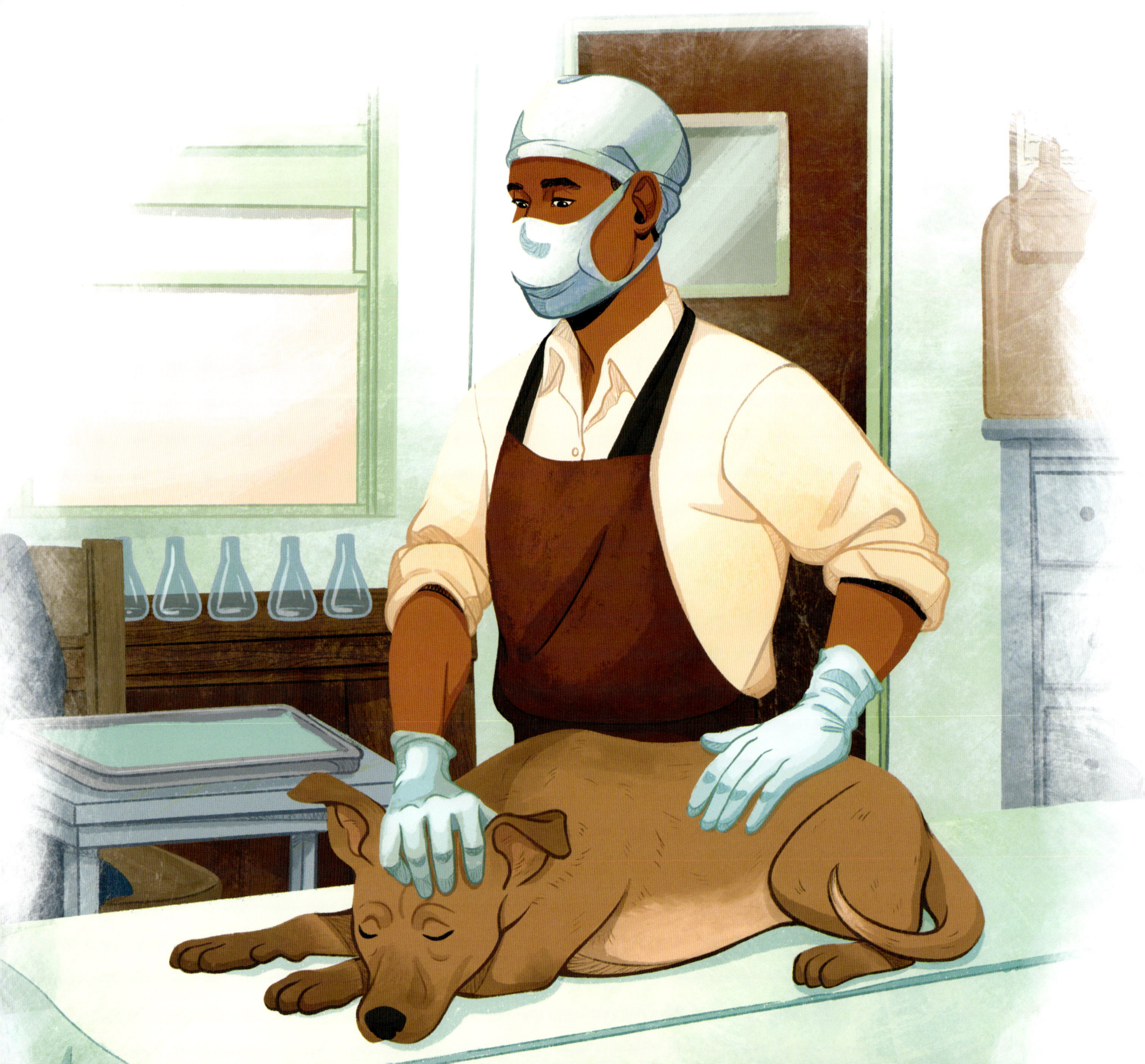

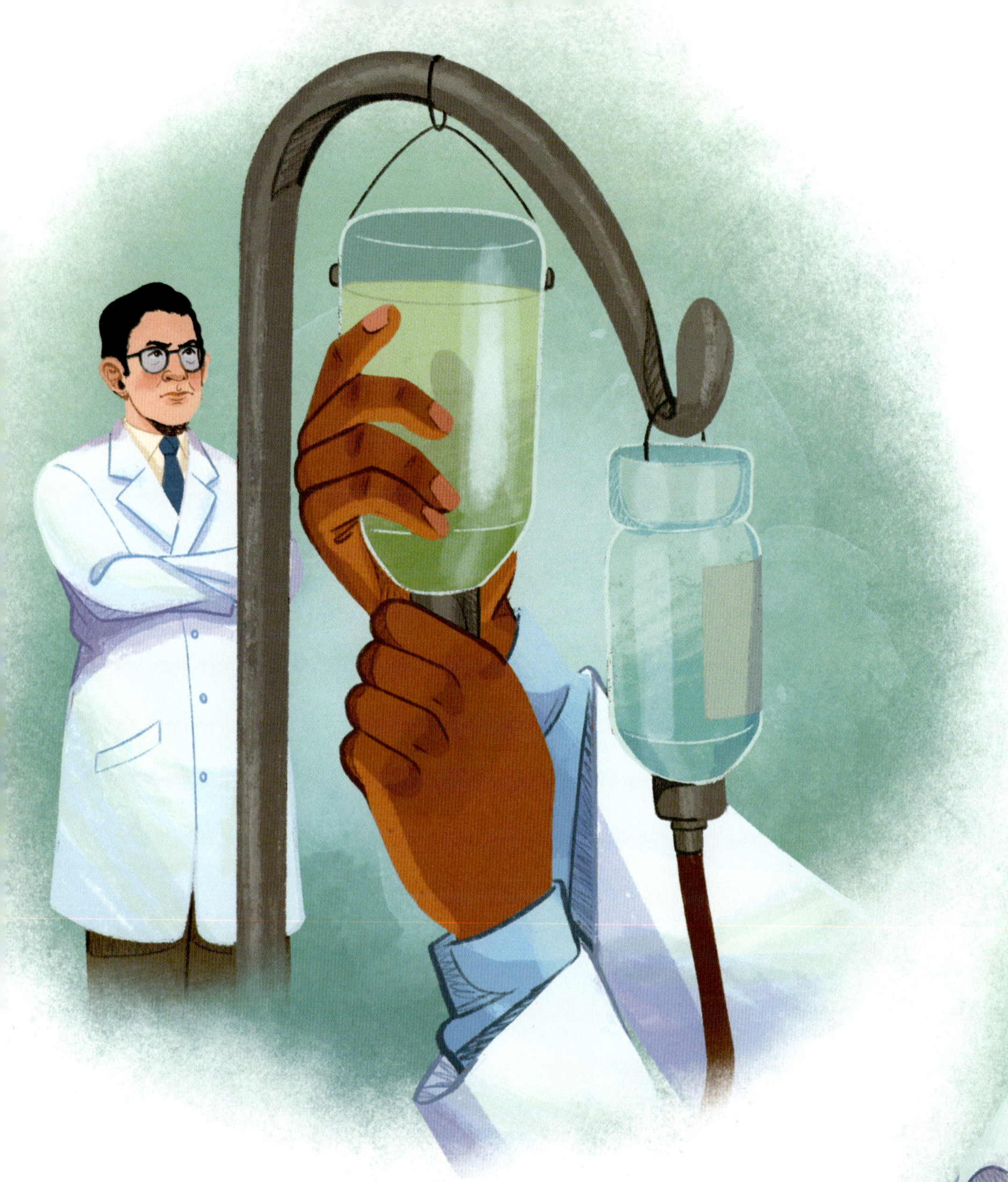

Once, when Vivien made an error, Dr. Blalock yelled at him. Vivien had been taught never to talk like that or to let someone talk to him in that way.

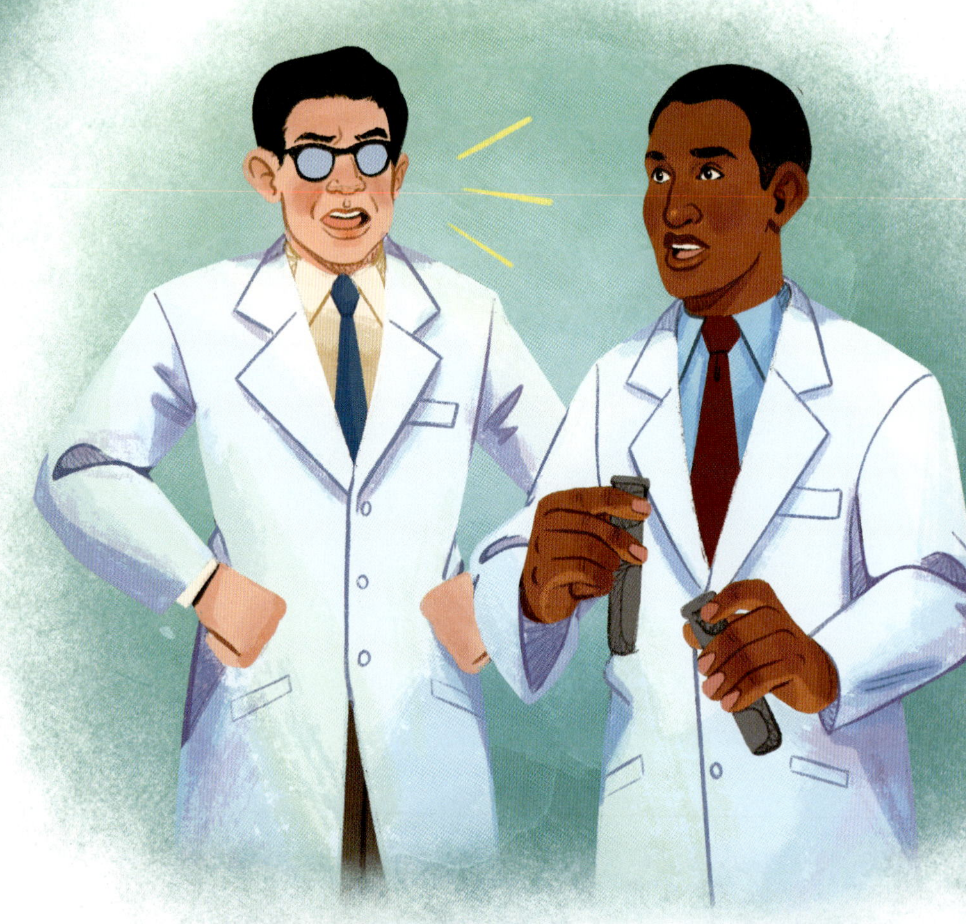

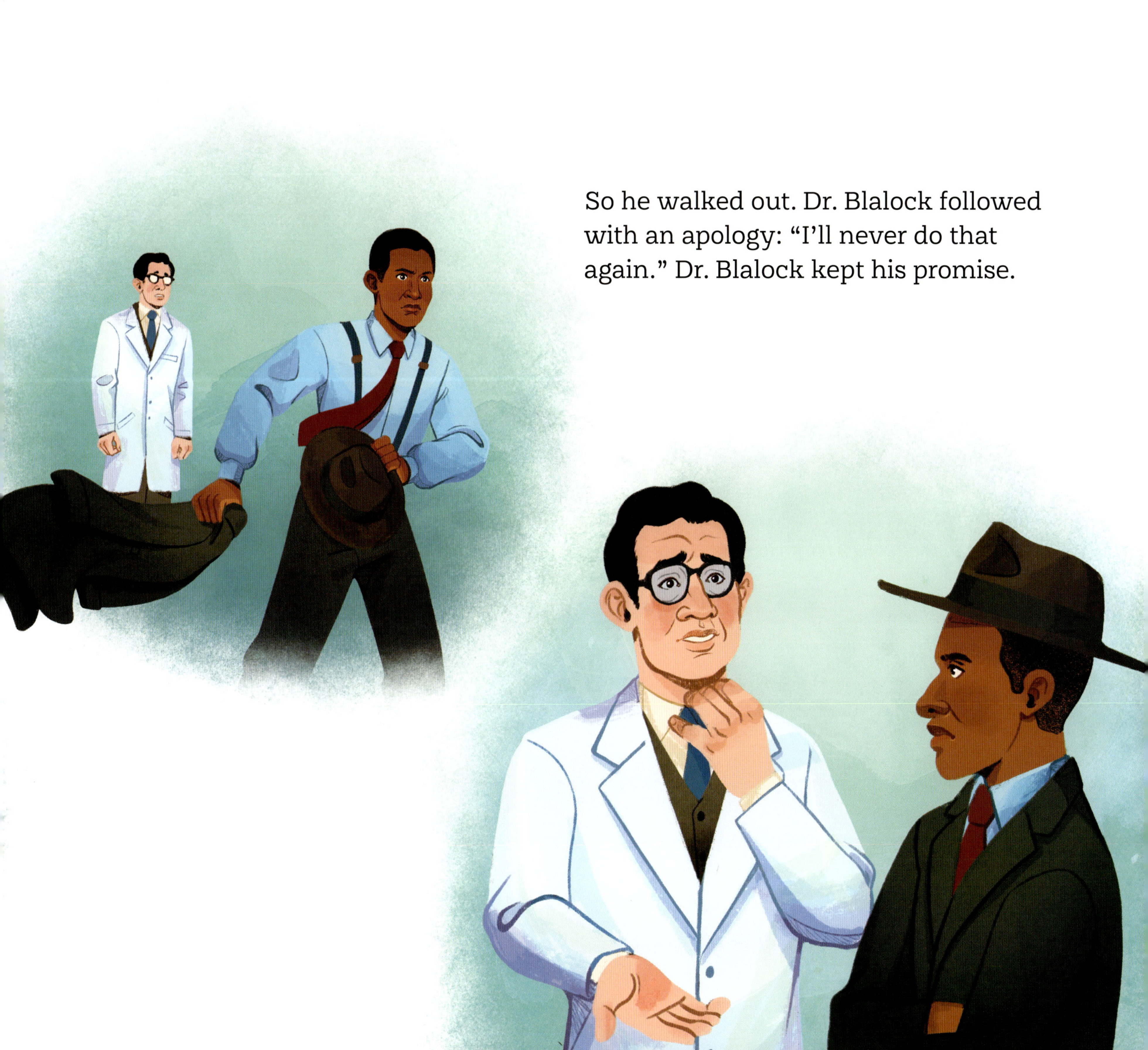

So he walked out. Dr. Blalock followed with an apology: “I’ll never do that again.” Dr. Blalock kept his promise.

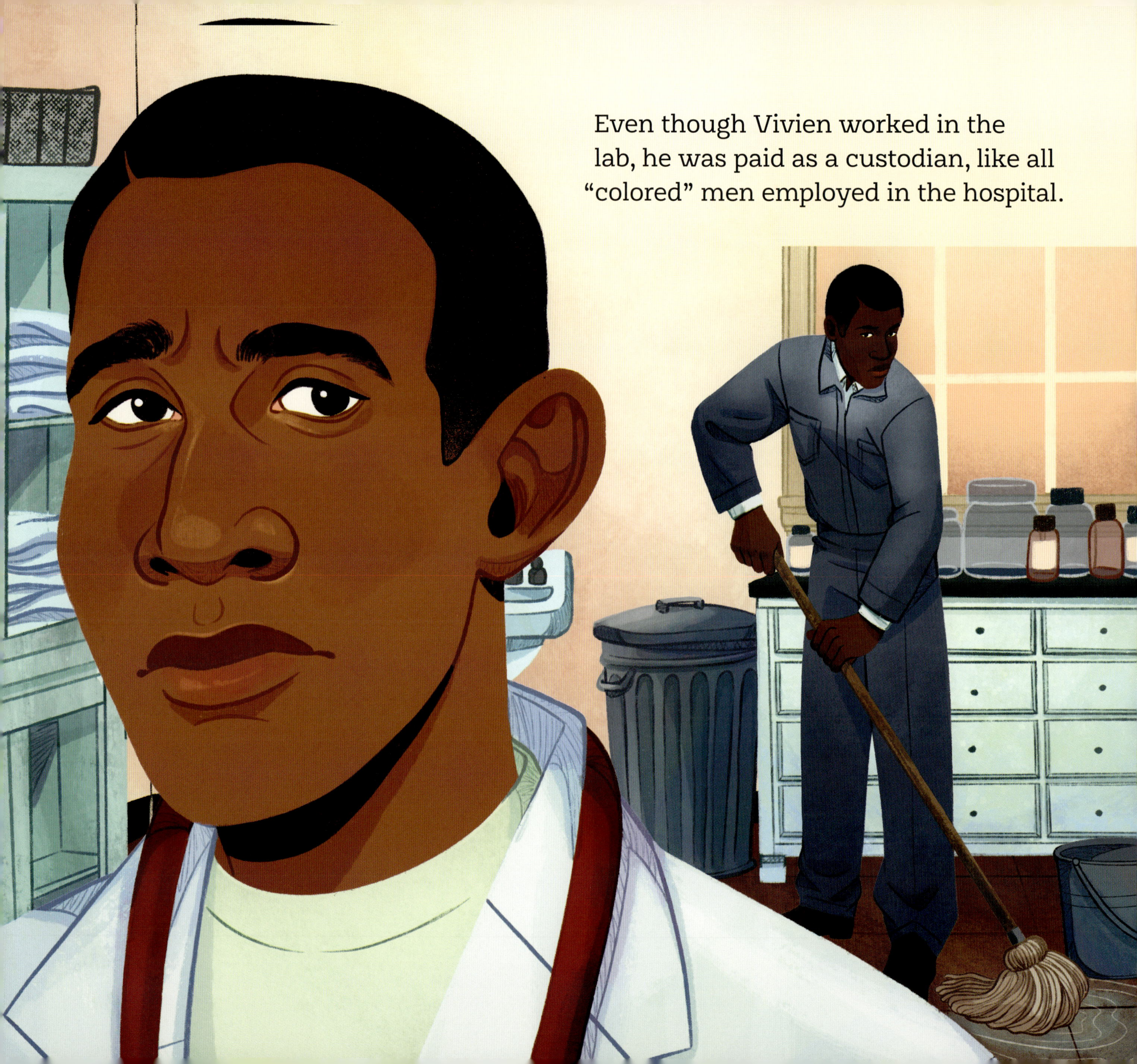

Even though Vivien worked in the lab, he was paid as a custodian, like all "colored" men employed in the hospital.

When Dr. Blalock learned Vivien was considering returning to his better-paying carpentry job, he arranged for a raise.

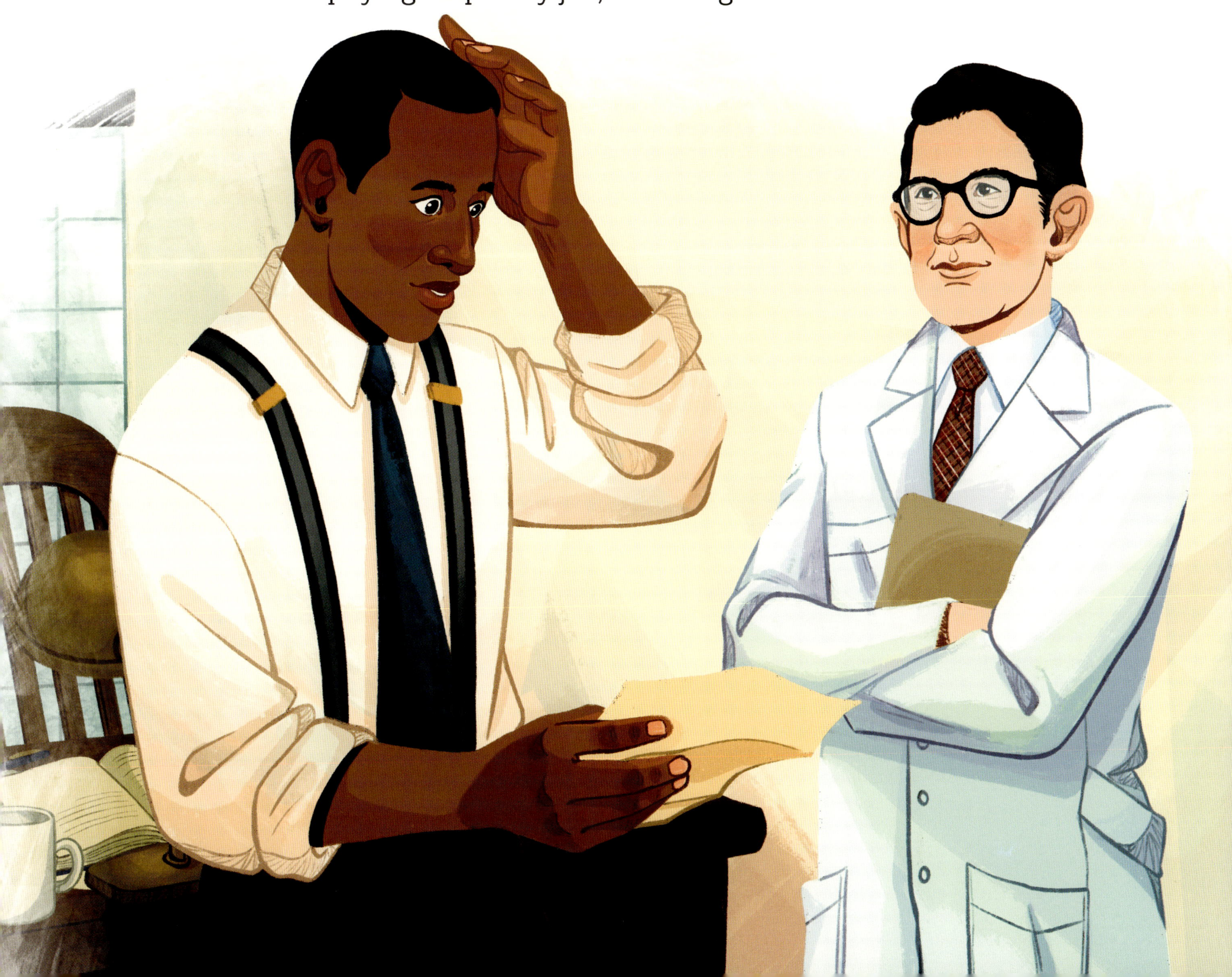

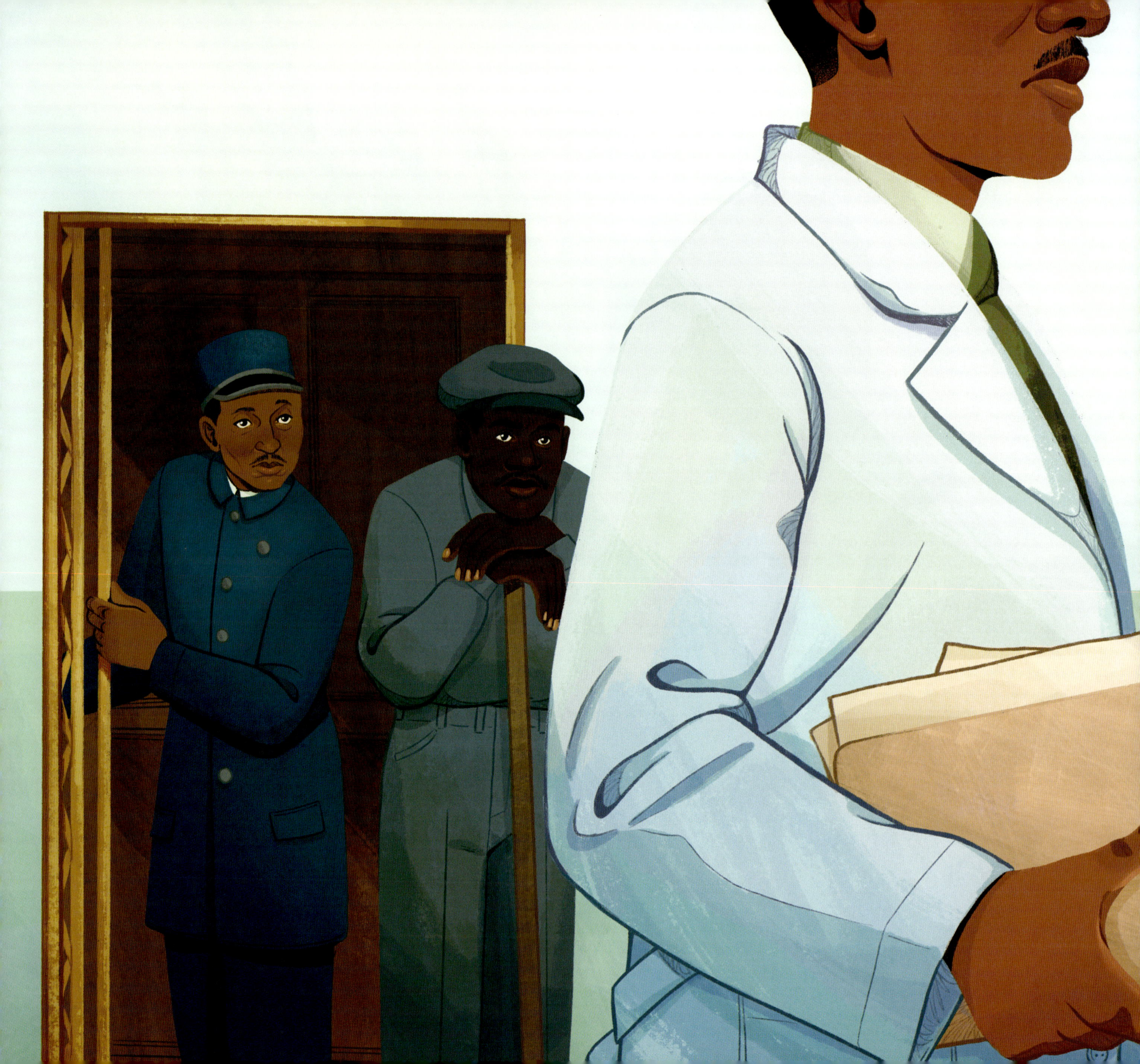

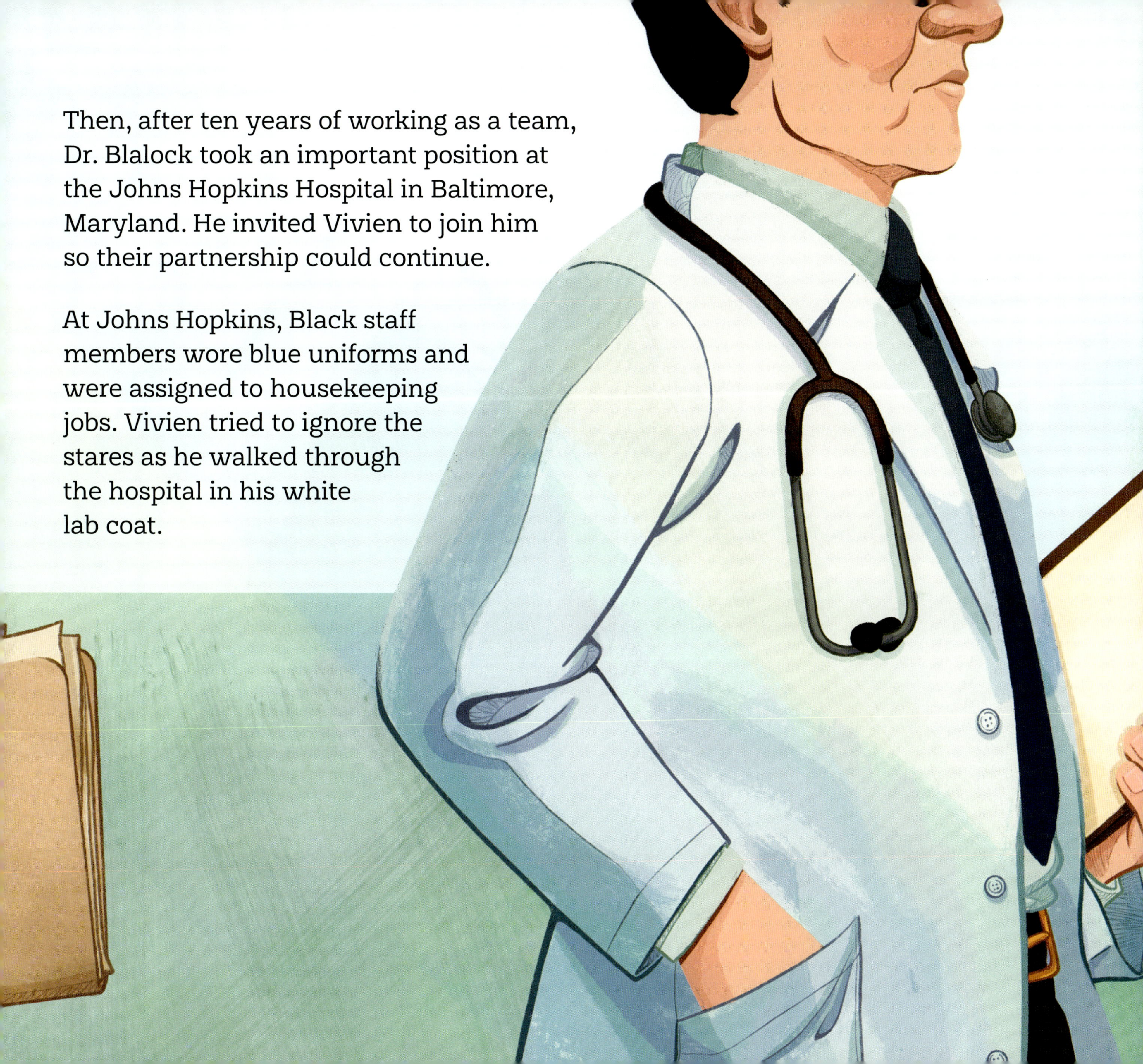

Then, after ten years of working as a team, Dr. Blalock took an important position at the Johns Hopkins Hospital in Baltimore, Maryland. He invited Vivien to join him so their partnership could continue.

At Johns Hopkins, Black staff members wore blue uniforms and were assigned to housekeeping jobs. Vivien tried to ignore the stares as he walked through the hospital in his white lab coat.

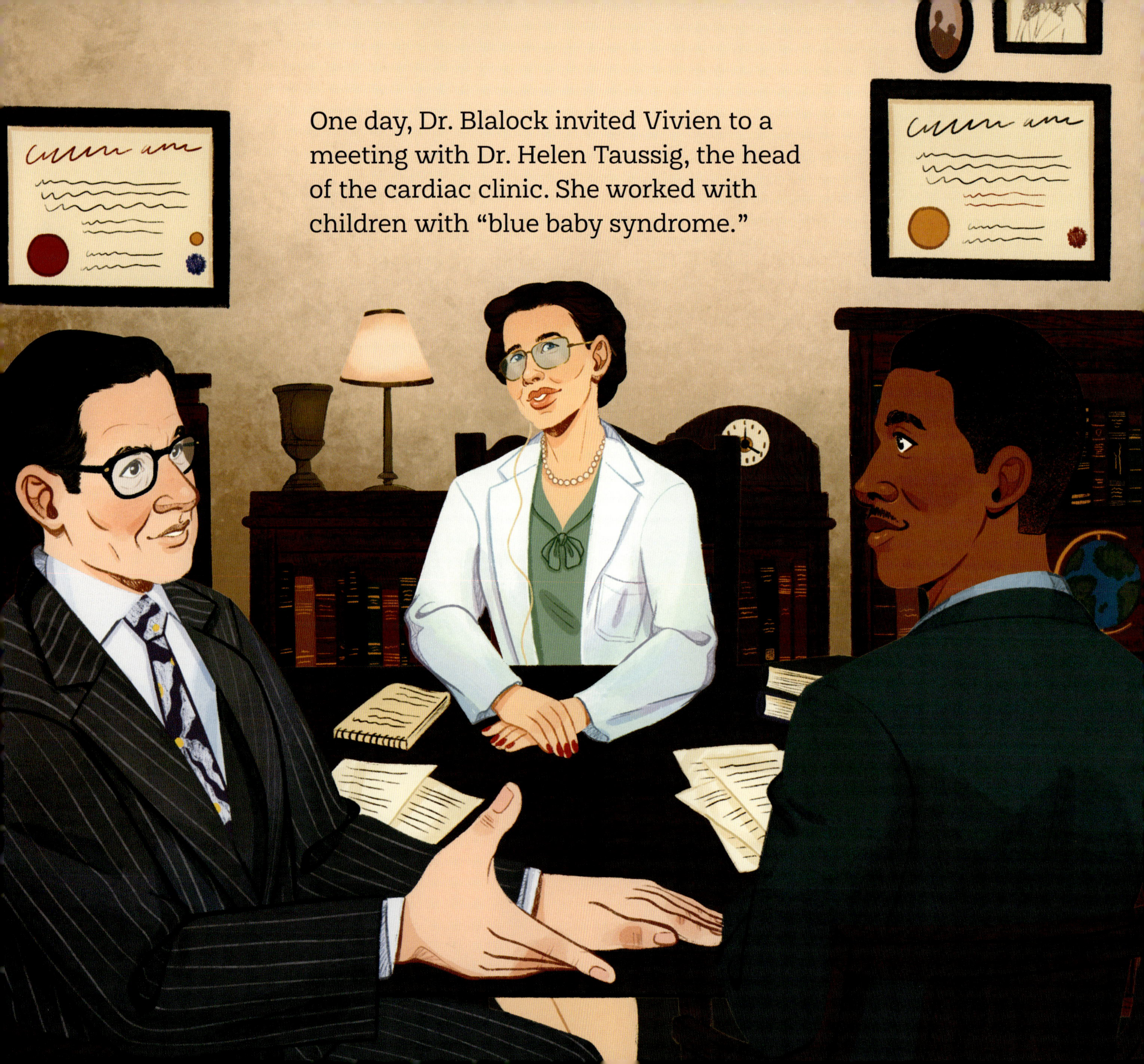

One day, Dr. Blalock invited Vivien to a meeting with Dr. Helen Taussig, the head of the cardiac clinic. She worked with children with “blue baby syndrome.”

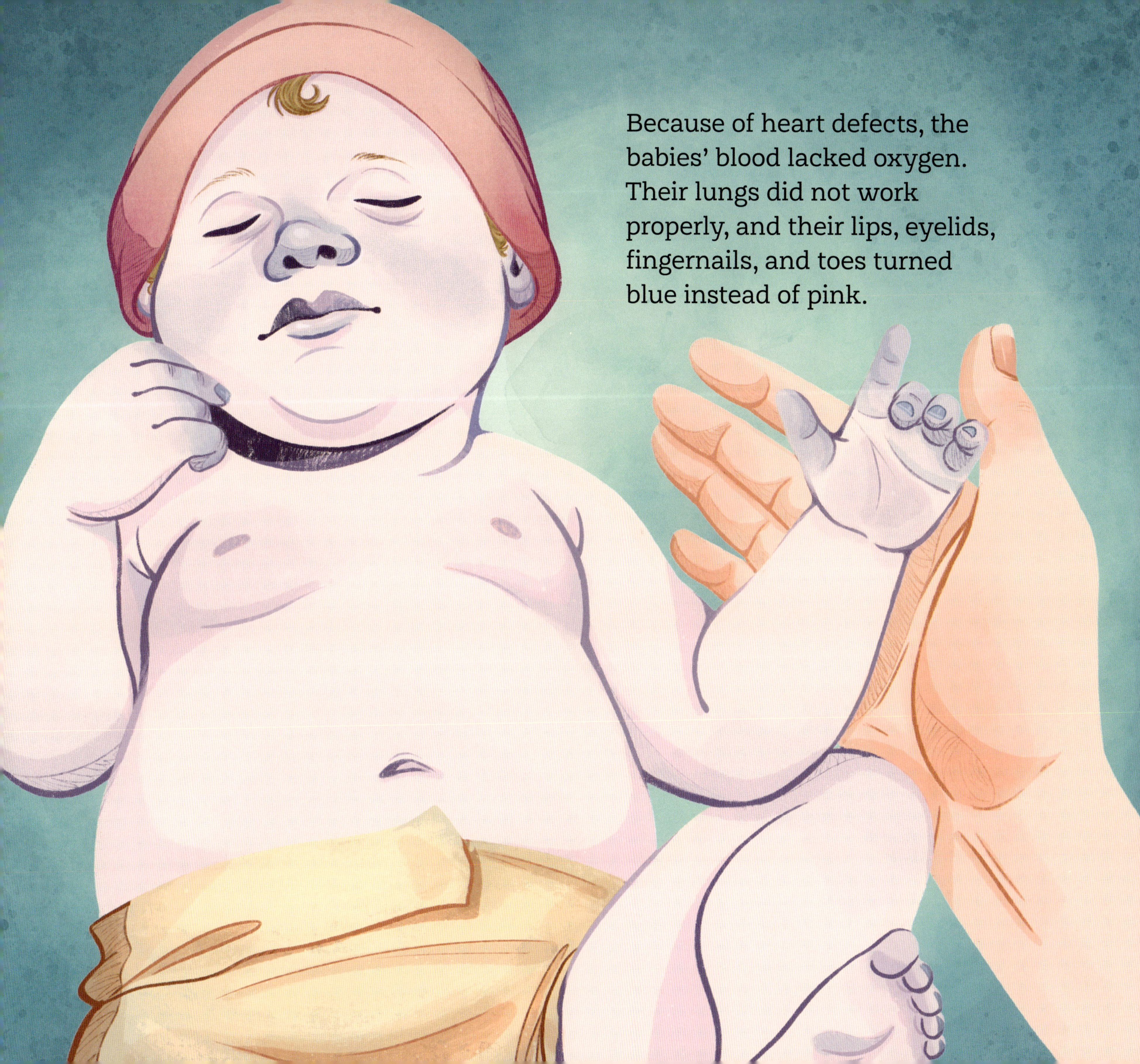

Because of heart defects, the babies' blood lacked oxygen. Their lungs did not work properly, and their lips, eyelids, fingernails, and toes turned blue instead of pink.

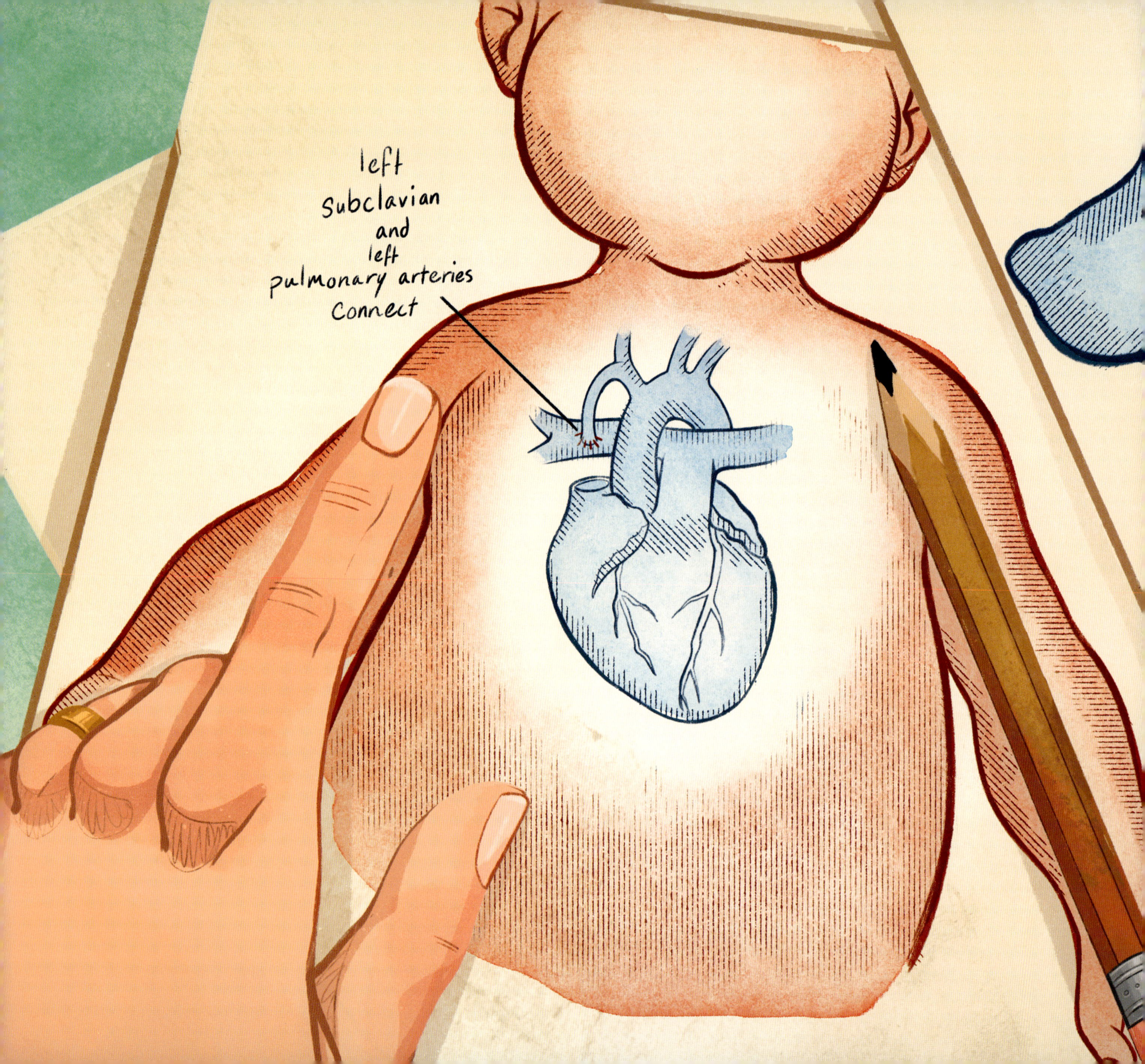
left
Subclavian
and
left
pulmonary arteries
Connect

Together, Dr. Blalock and Vivien designed a way to reroute the blood from the heart to the lungs, increasing the flow of oxygen to the blood. To test the technique, Vivien created blue baby–like conditions in dogs and then corrected the problem.

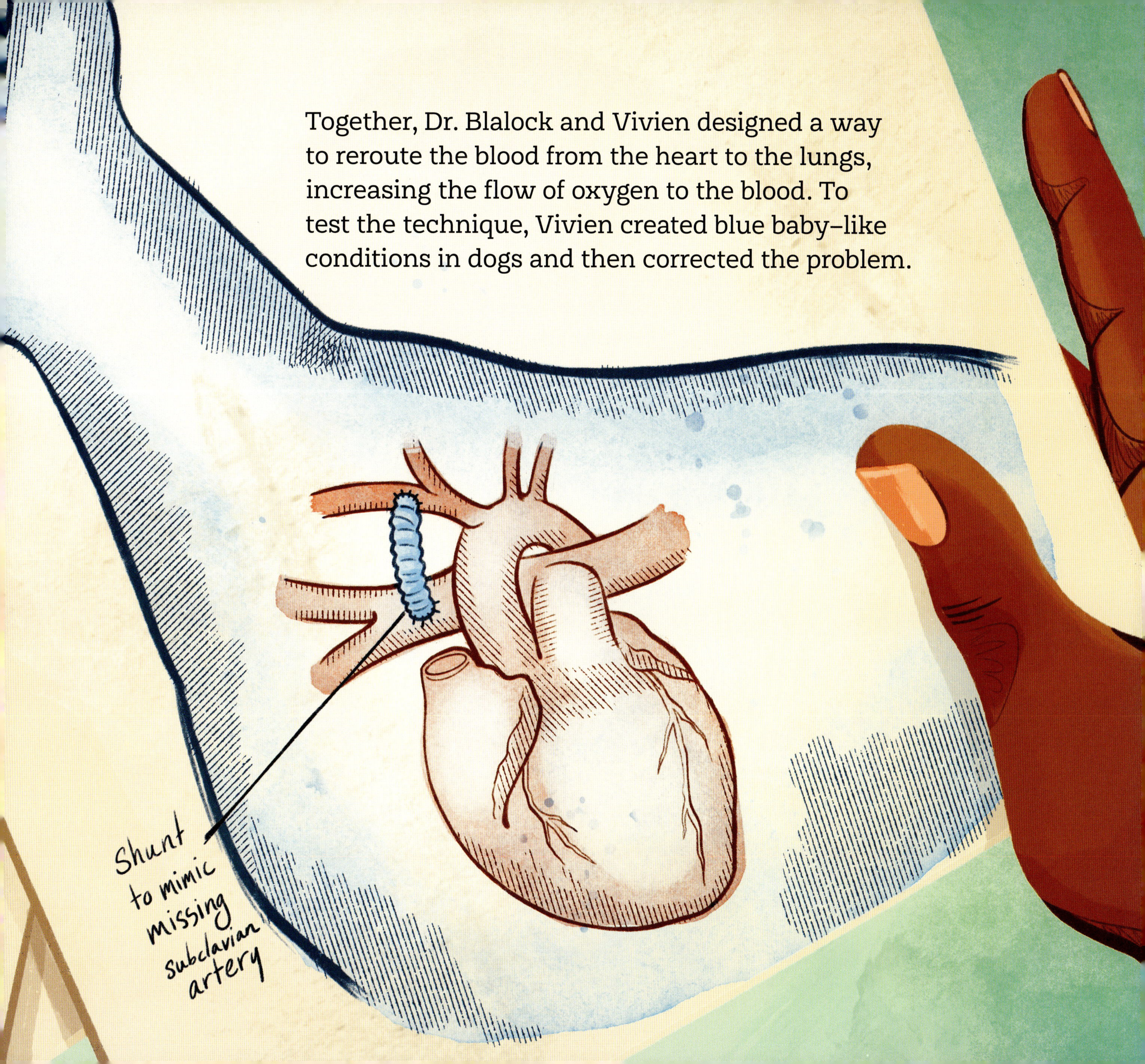

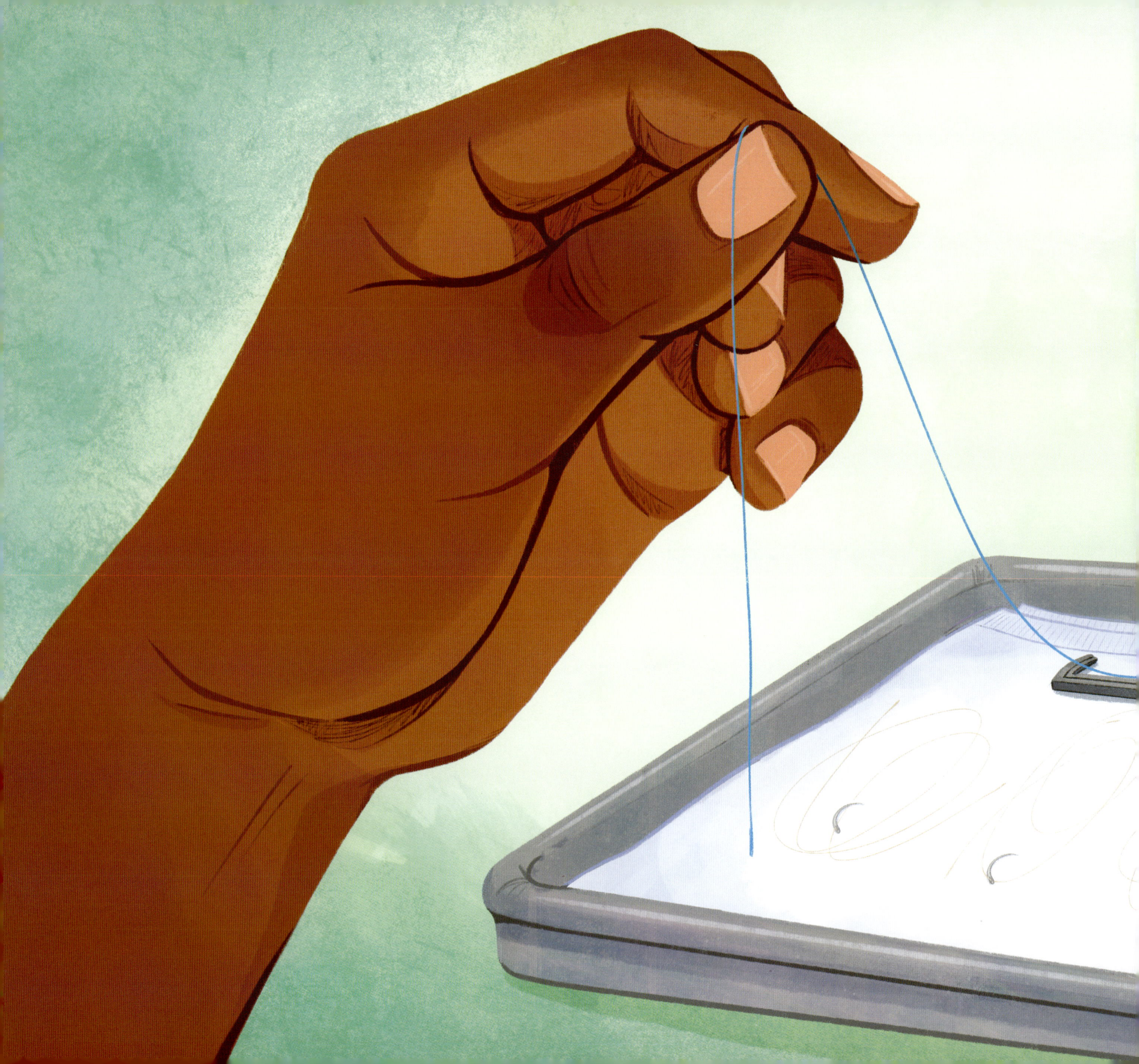

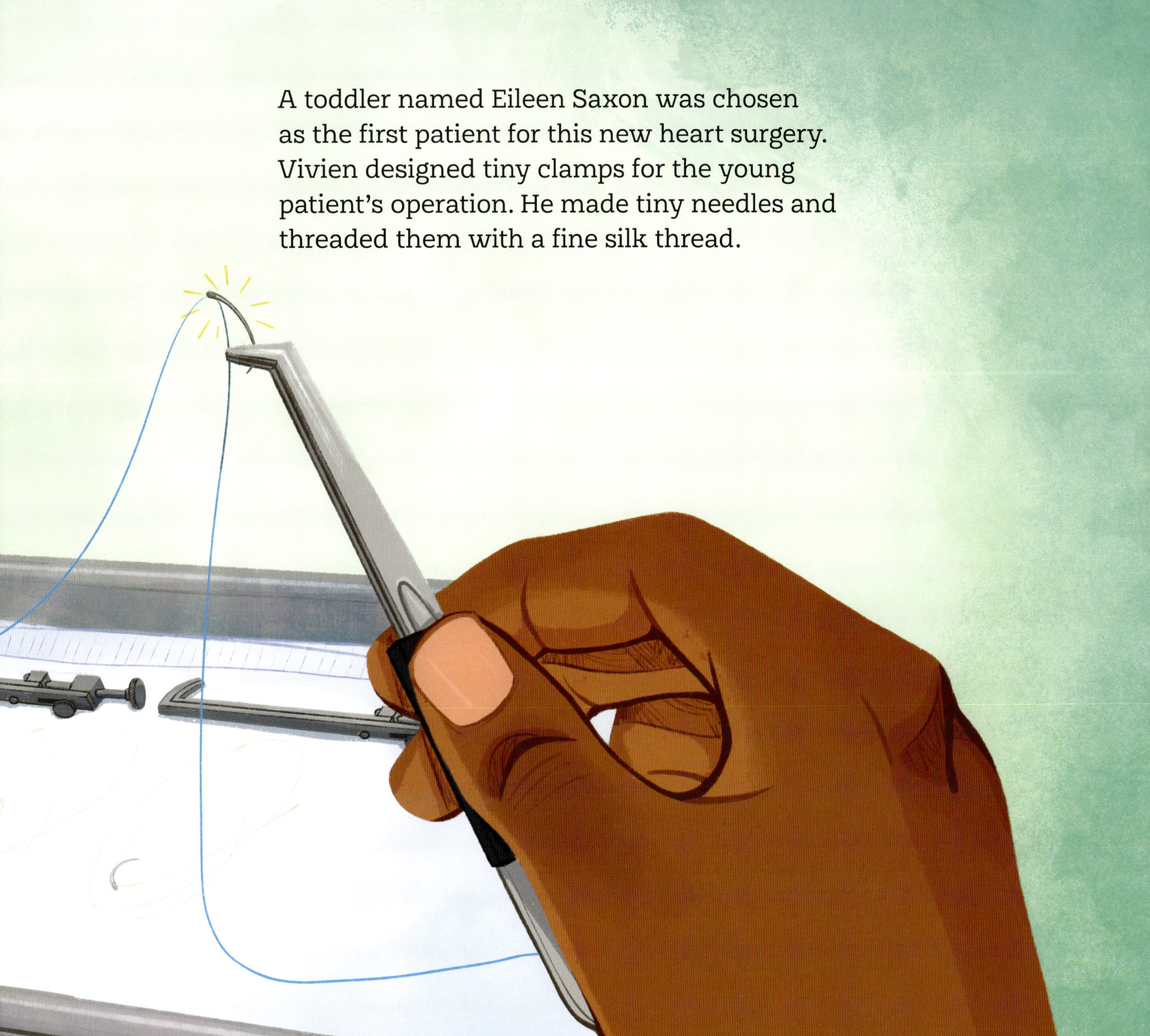

A toddler named Eileen Saxon was chosen as the first patient for this new heart surgery. Vivien designed tiny clamps for the young patient's operation. He made tiny needles and threaded them with a fine silk thread.

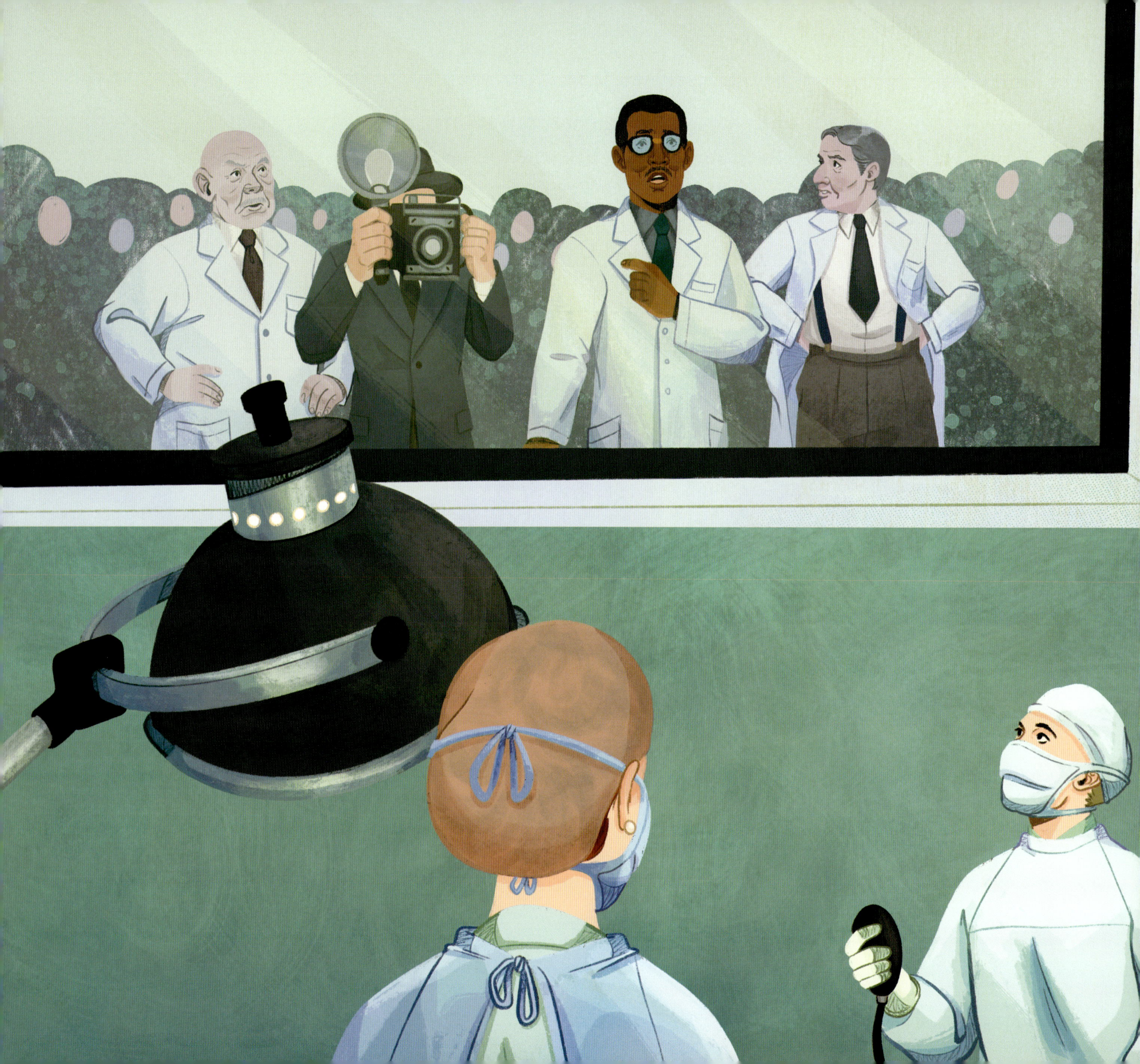

When it was time for the surgery, Vivien went to the gallery above the operating room to watch. In those days, only white doctors and nurses were allowed in the operating room with white patients. Vivien had performed the surgery hundreds of times on dogs. Dr. Blalock had done so only once.

"Vivien, you'd better come down here," said Dr. Blalock.

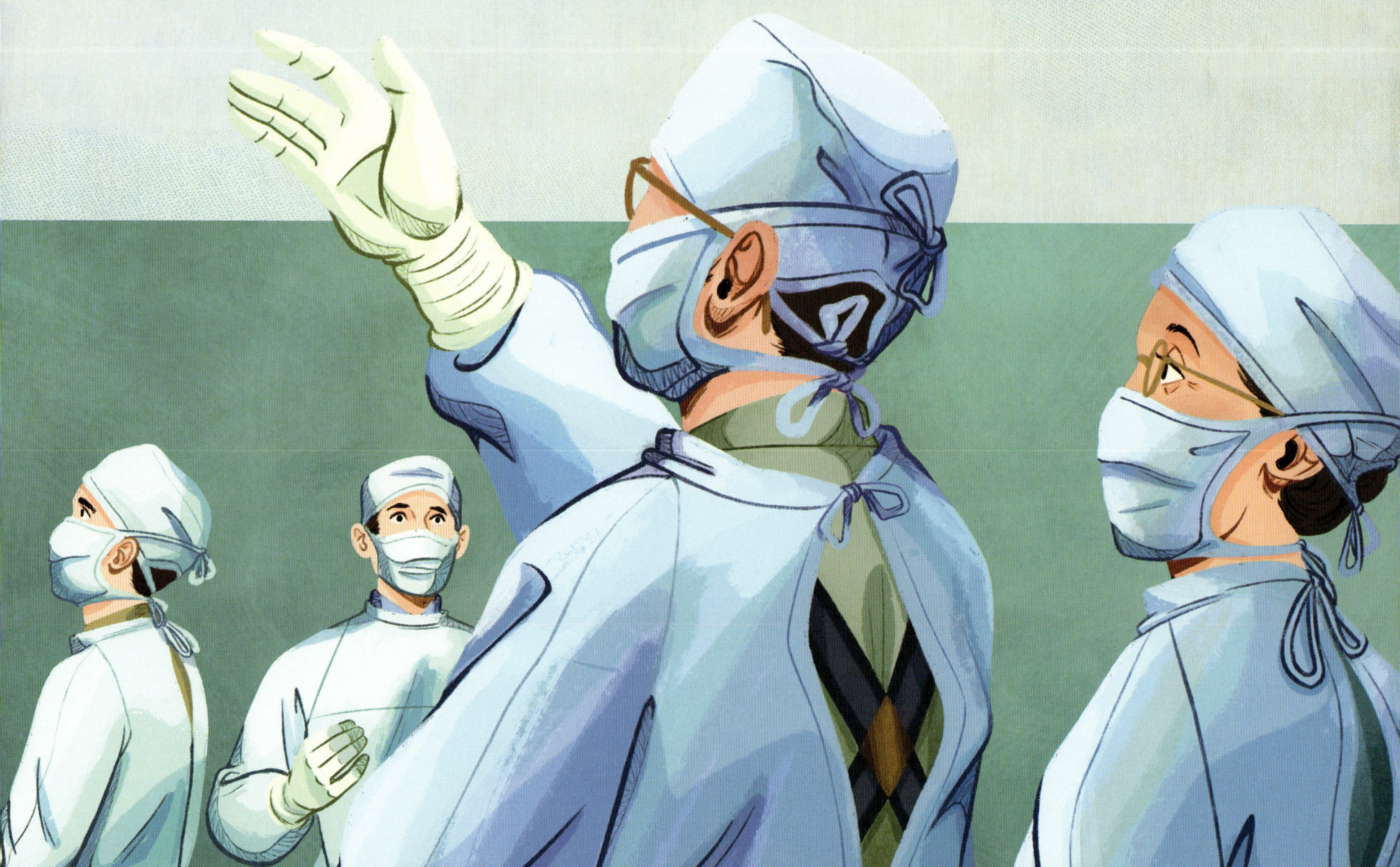

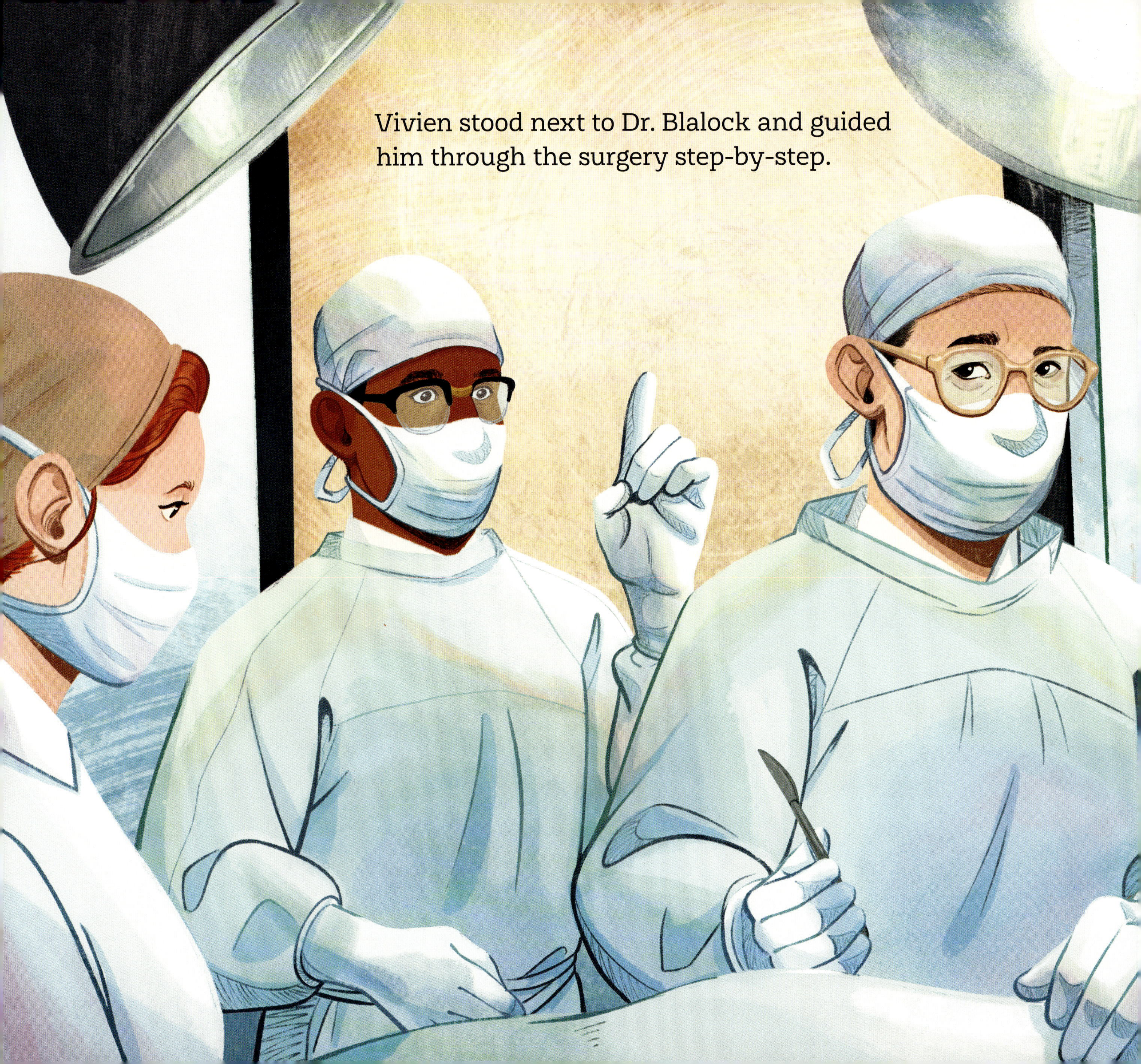

Vivien stood next to Dr. Blalock and guided him through the surgery step-by-step.

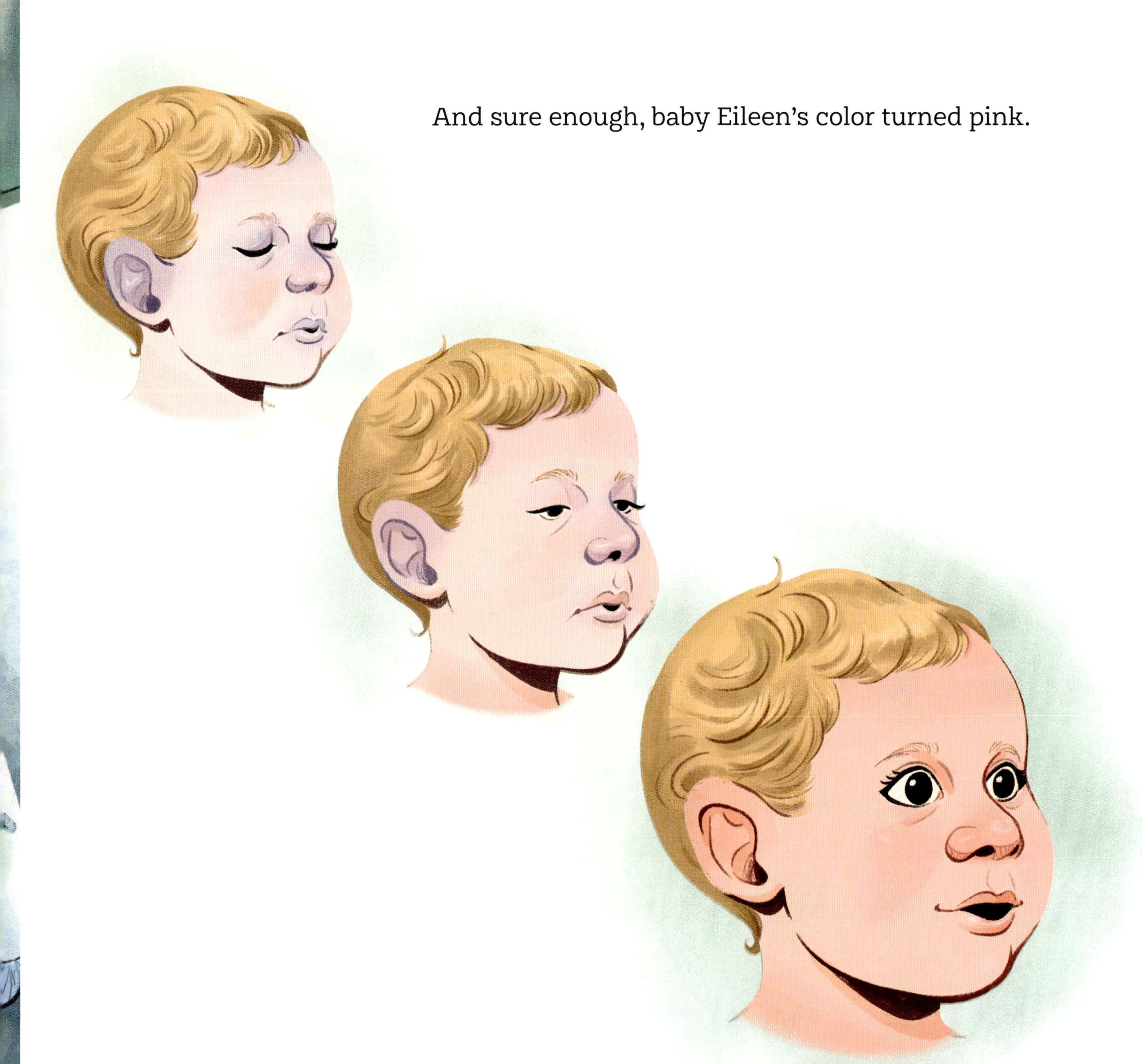

And sure enough, baby Eileen's color turned pink.

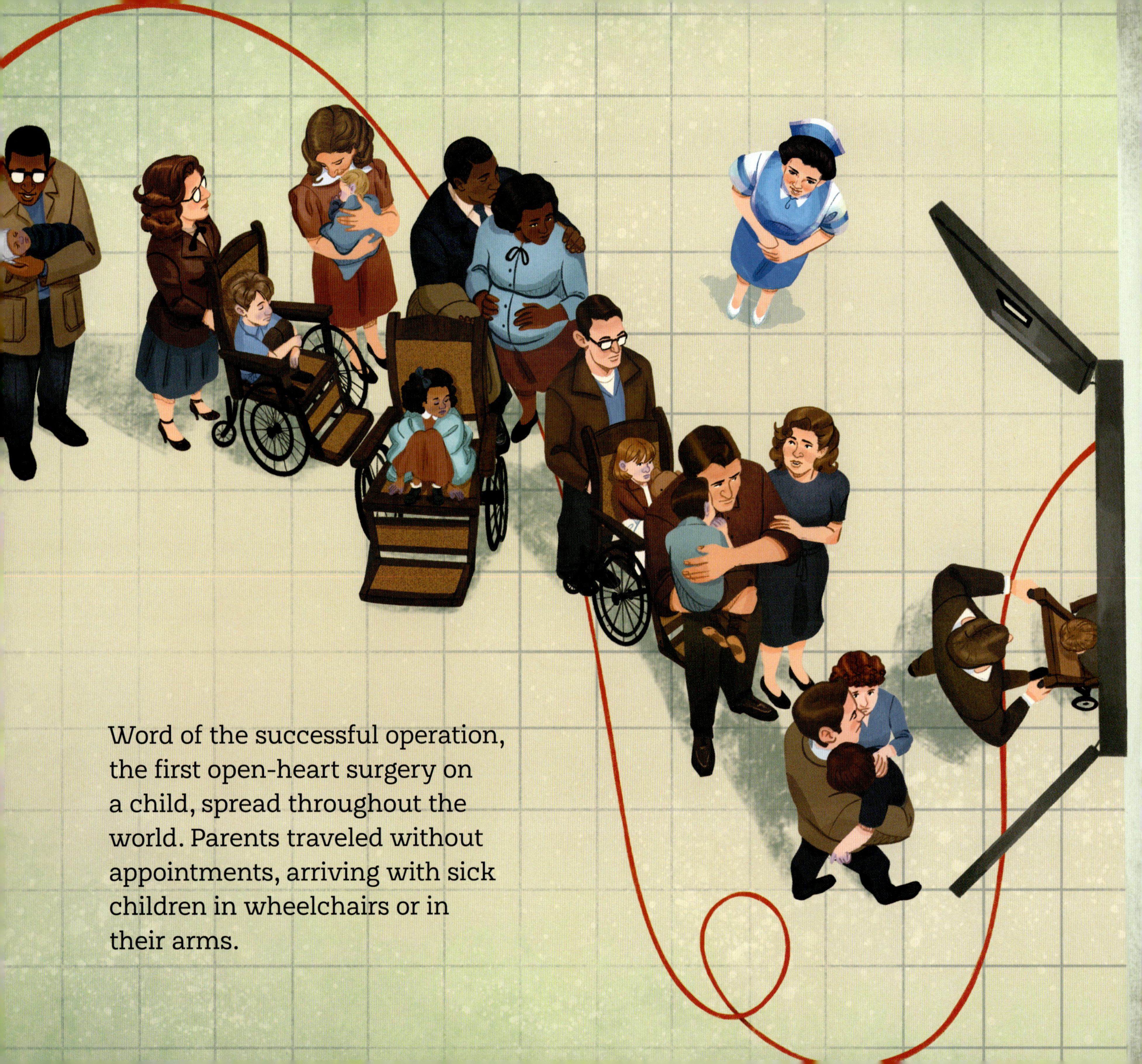

Word of the successful operation, the first open-heart surgery on a child, spread throughout the world. Parents traveled without appointments, arriving with sick children in wheelchairs or in their arms.

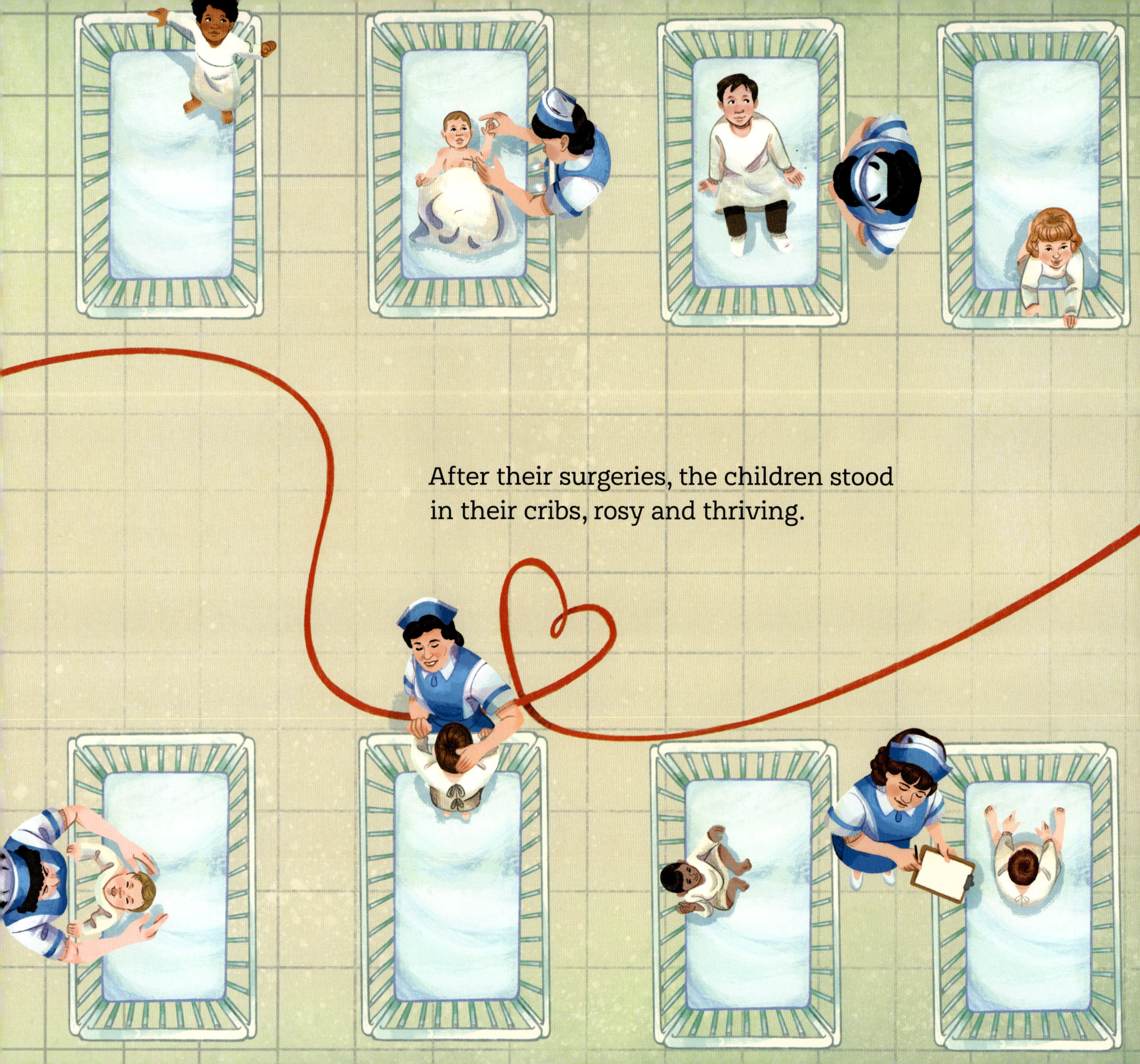

After their surgeries, the children stood
in their cribs, rosy and thriving.

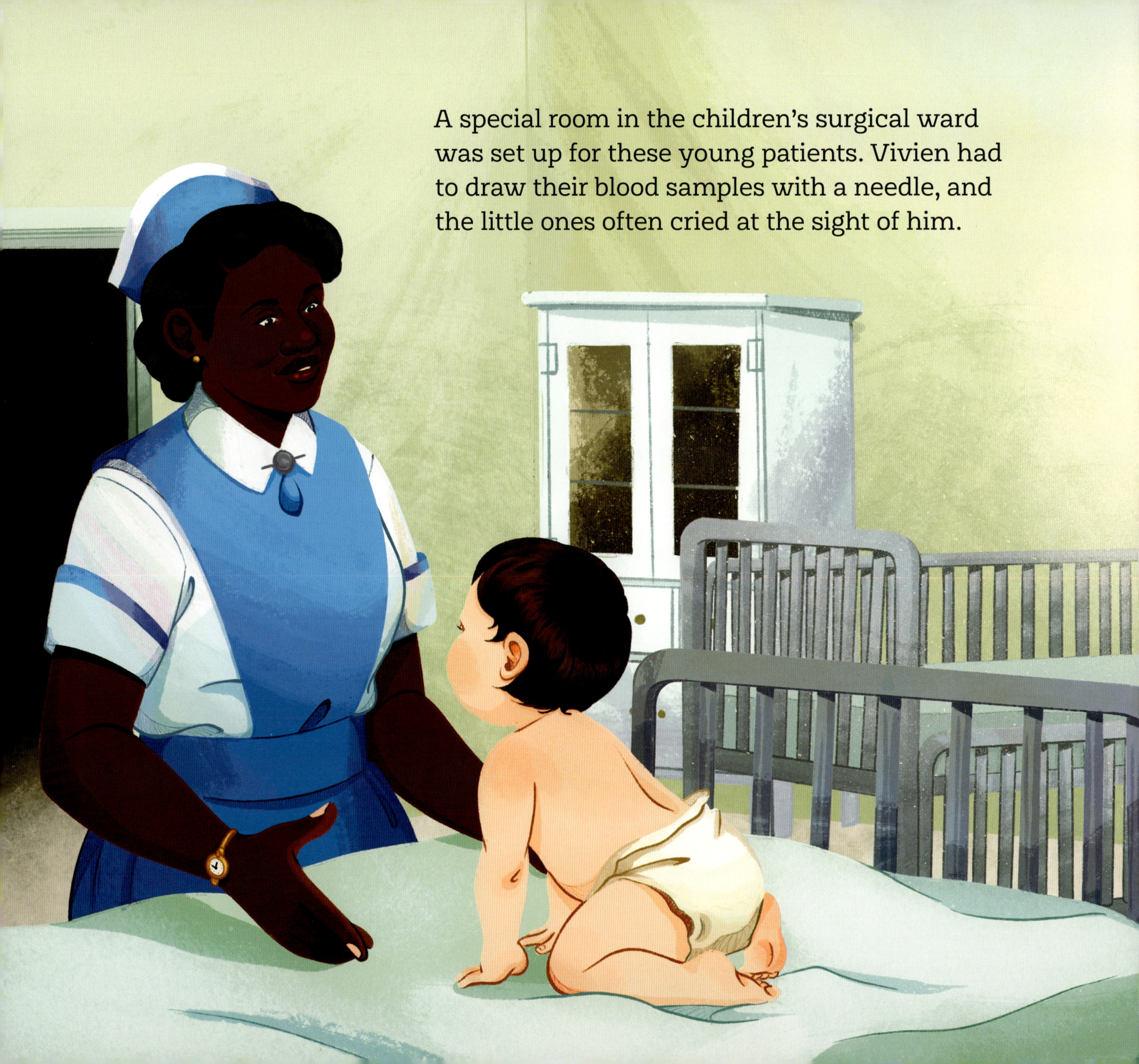

A special room in the children's surgical ward was set up for these young patients. Vivien had to draw their blood samples with a needle, and the little ones often cried at the sight of him.

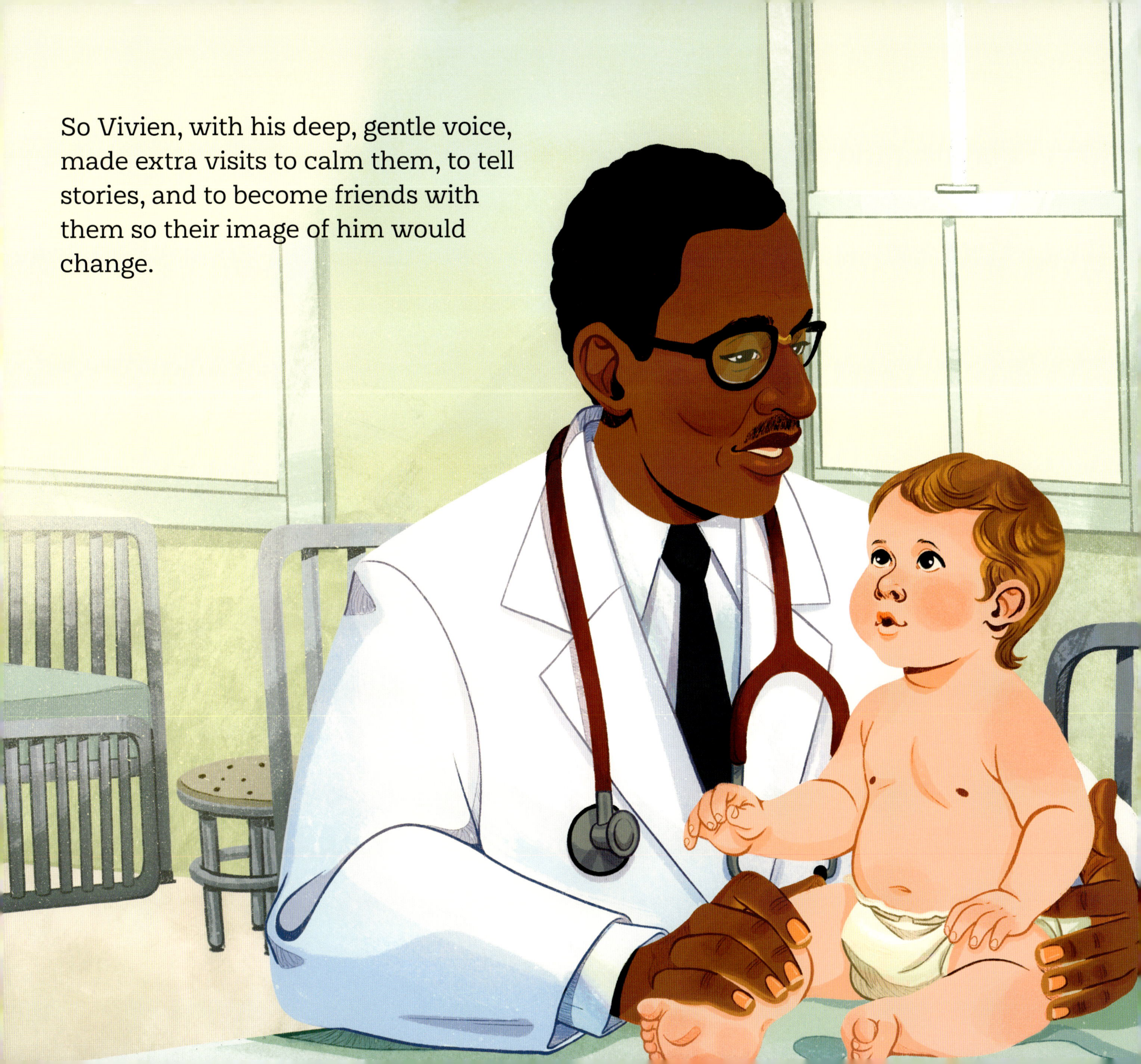

So Vivien, with his deep, gentle voice, made extra visits to calm them, to tell stories, and to become friends with them so their image of him would change.

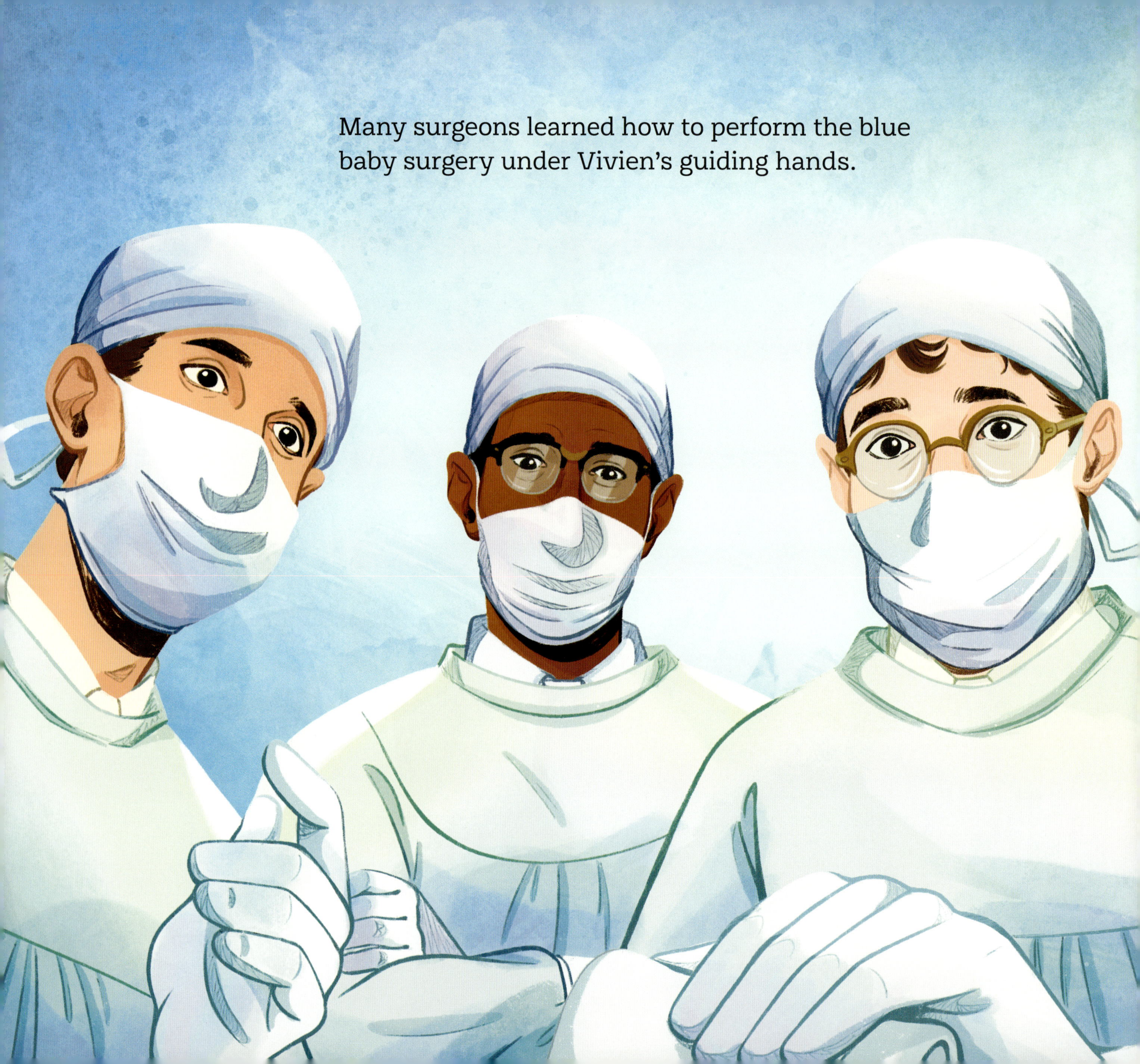

Many surgeons learned how to perform the blue baby surgery under Vivien's guiding hands.

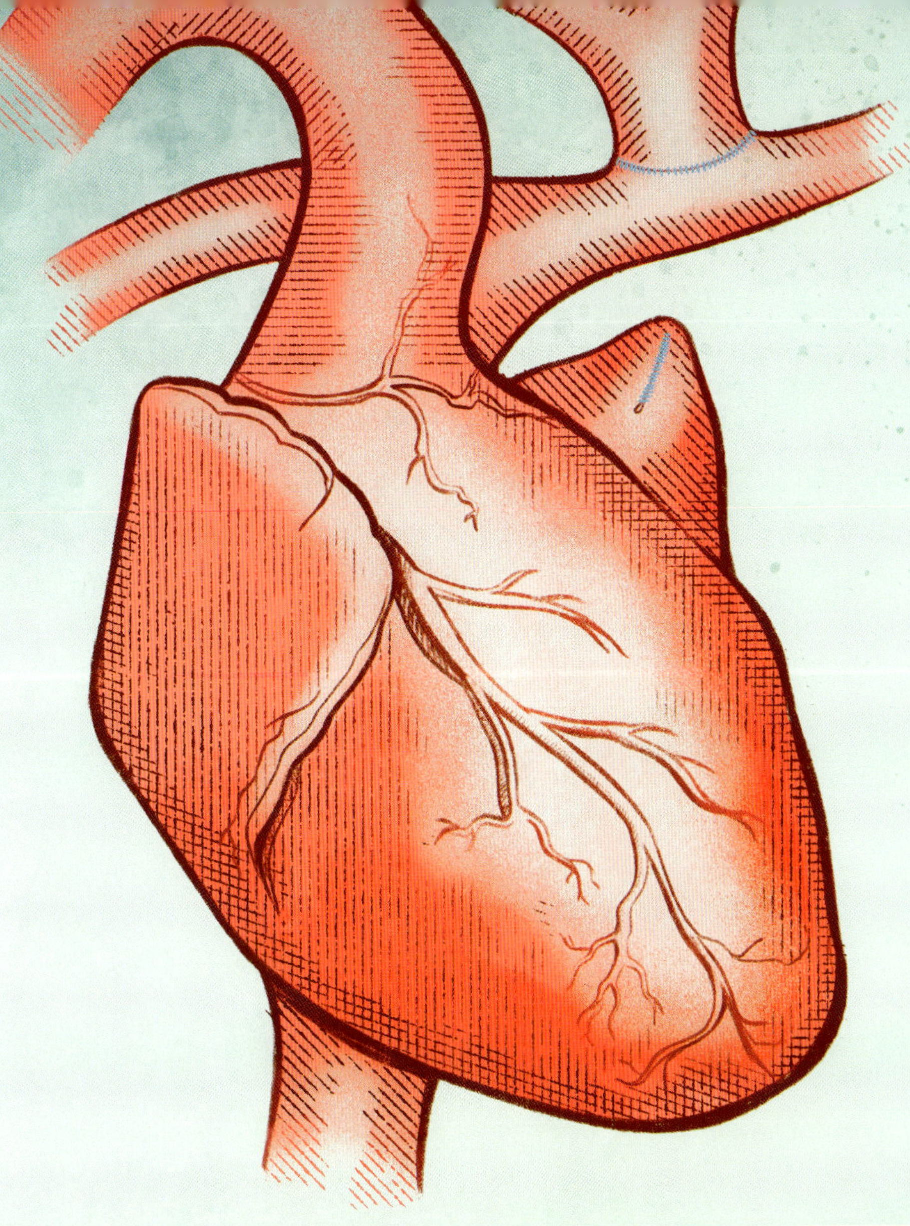

One day, Dr. Blalock examined an almost invisible line of stitches.

"Vivien, are you sure you did this?" asked Dr. Blalock.

Vivien nodded.

"This looks like something the Lord made," said Dr. Blalock.

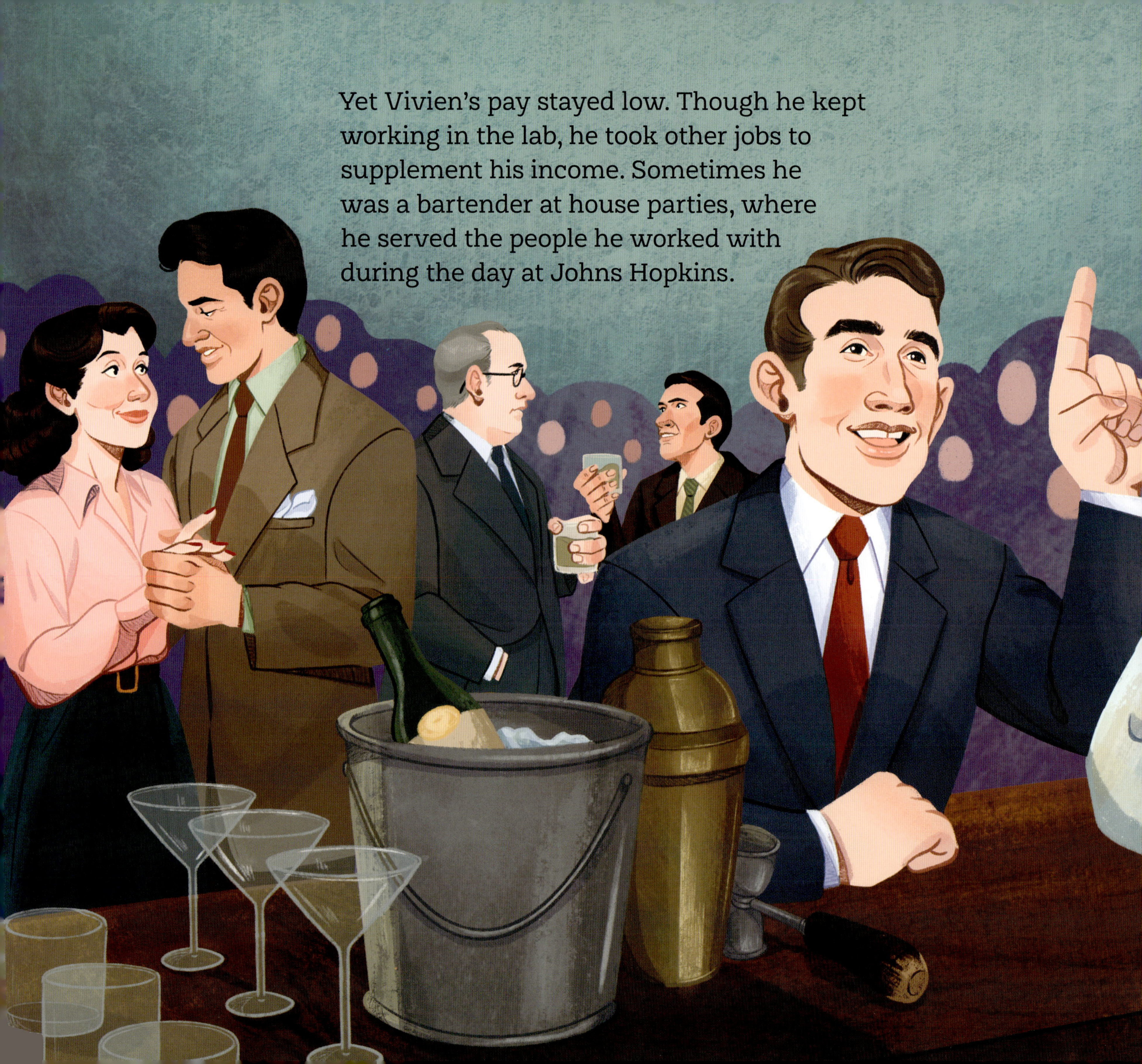

Yet Vivien's pay stayed low. Though he kept working in the lab, he took other jobs to supplement his income. Sometimes he was a bartender at house parties, where he served the people he worked with during the day at Johns Hopkins.

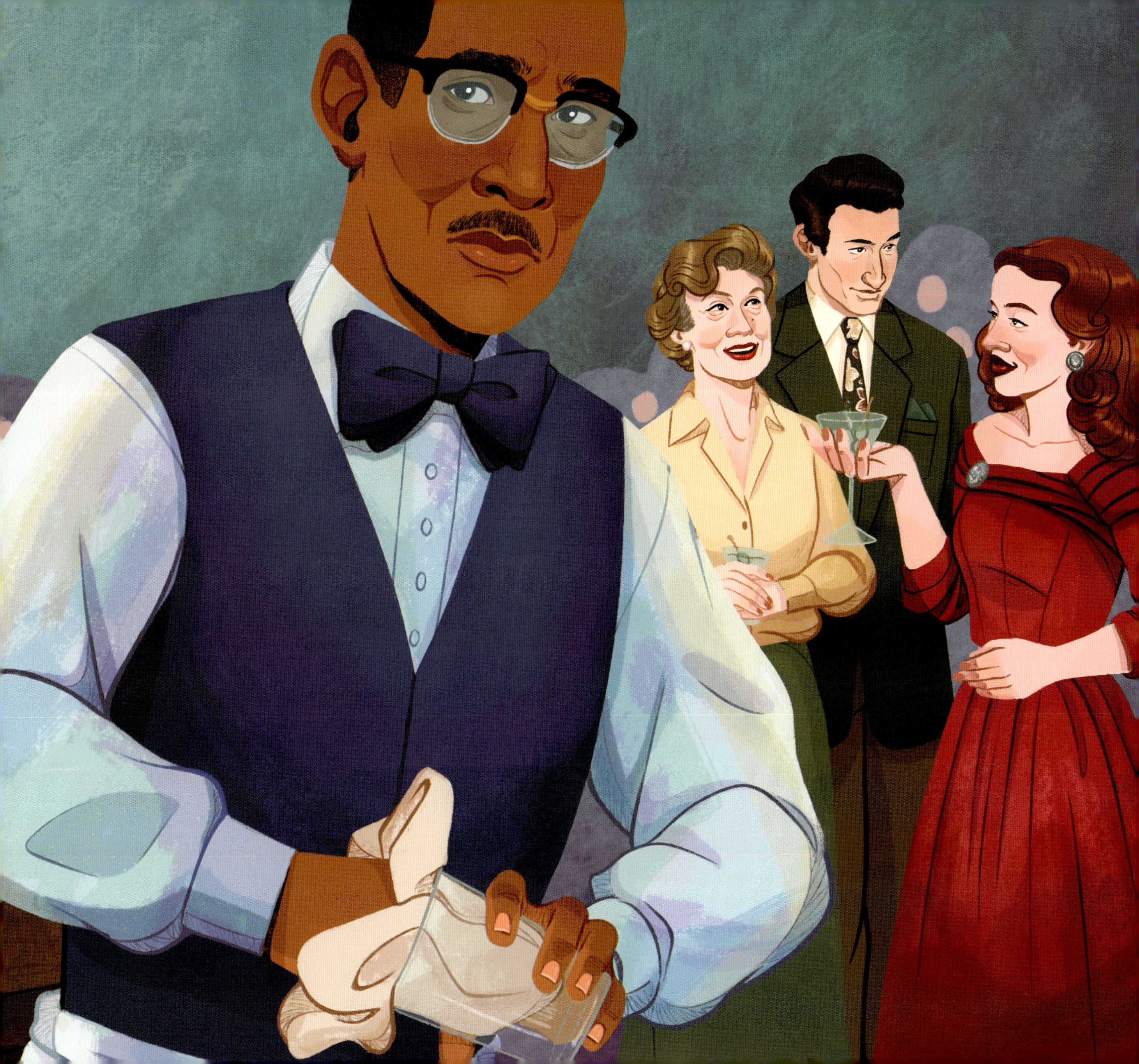

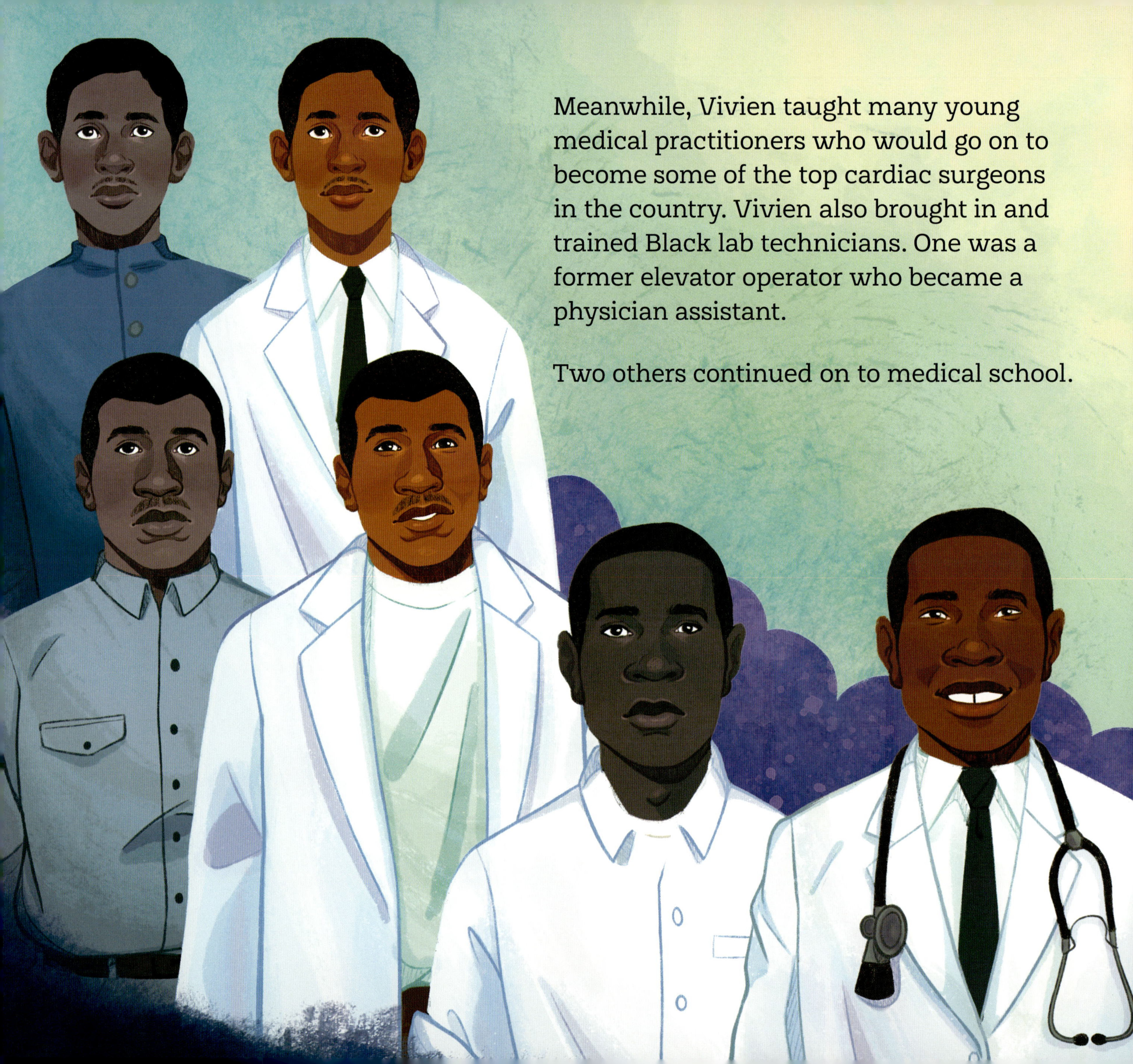

Meanwhile, Vivien taught many young medical practitioners who would go on to become some of the top cardiac surgeons in the country. Vivien also brought in and trained Black lab technicians. One was a former elevator operator who became a physician assistant.

Two others continued on to medical school.

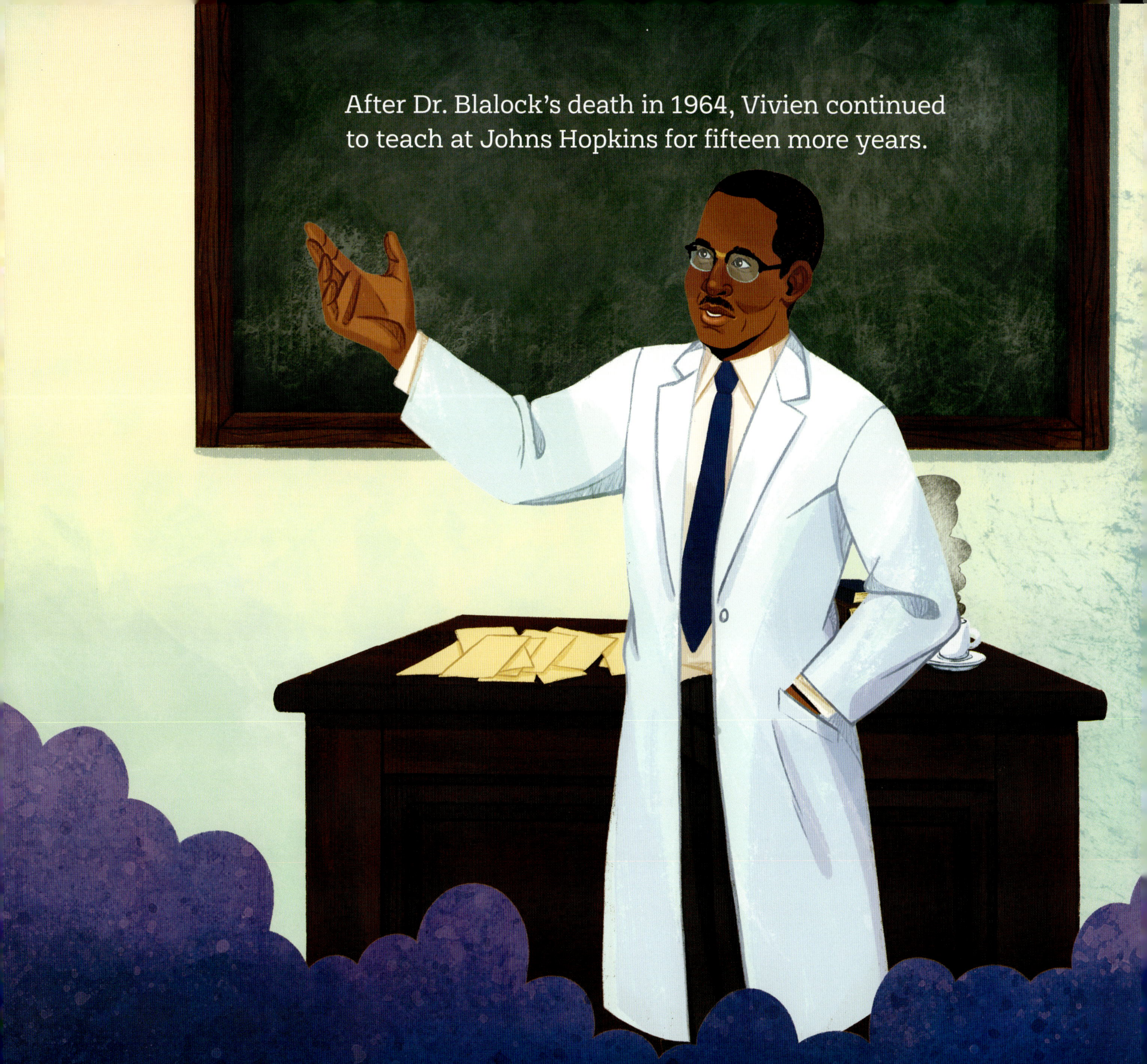

After Dr. Blalock's death in 1964, Vivien continued to teach at Johns Hopkins for fifteen more years.

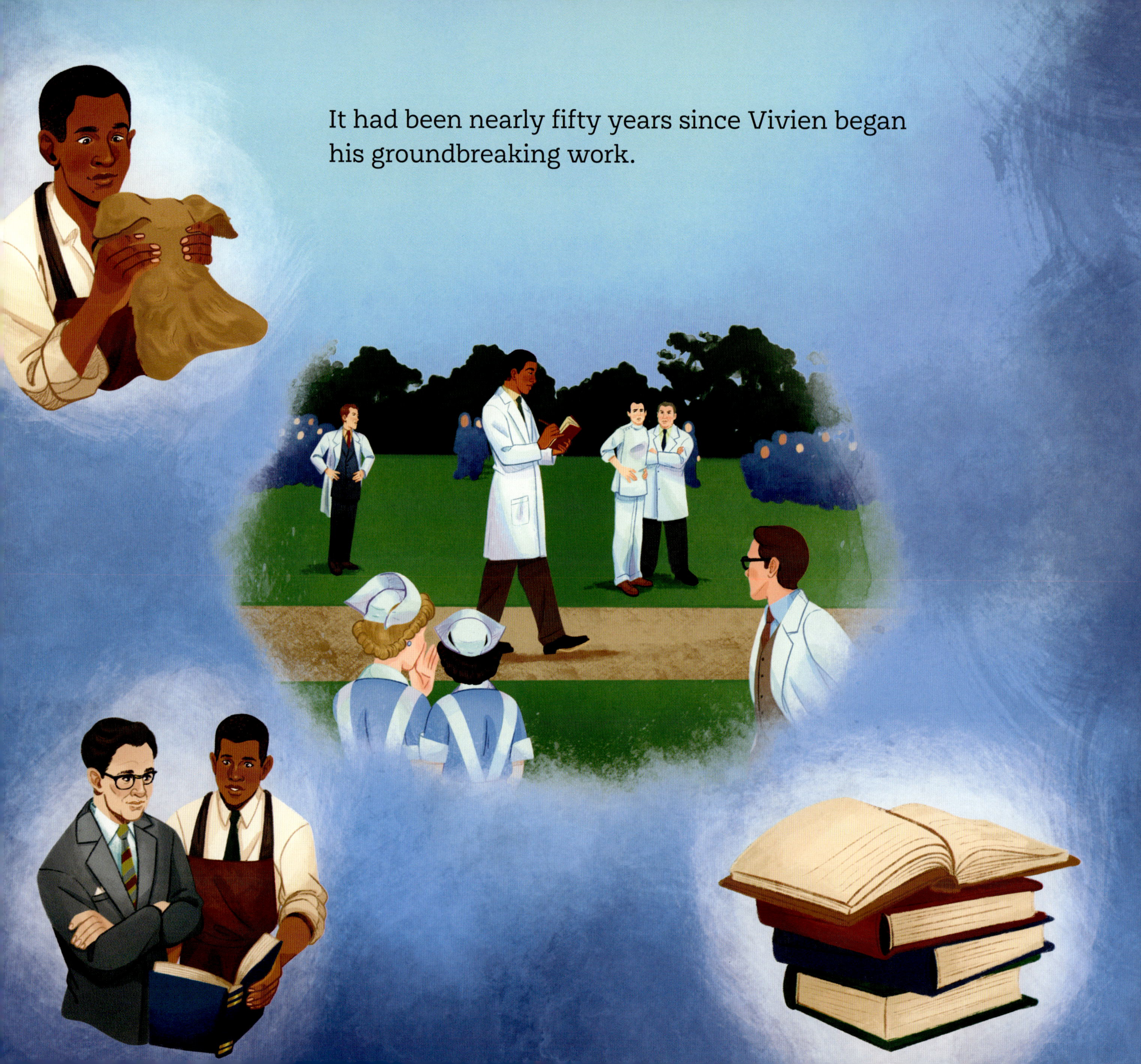

It had been nearly fifty years since Vivien began his groundbreaking work.

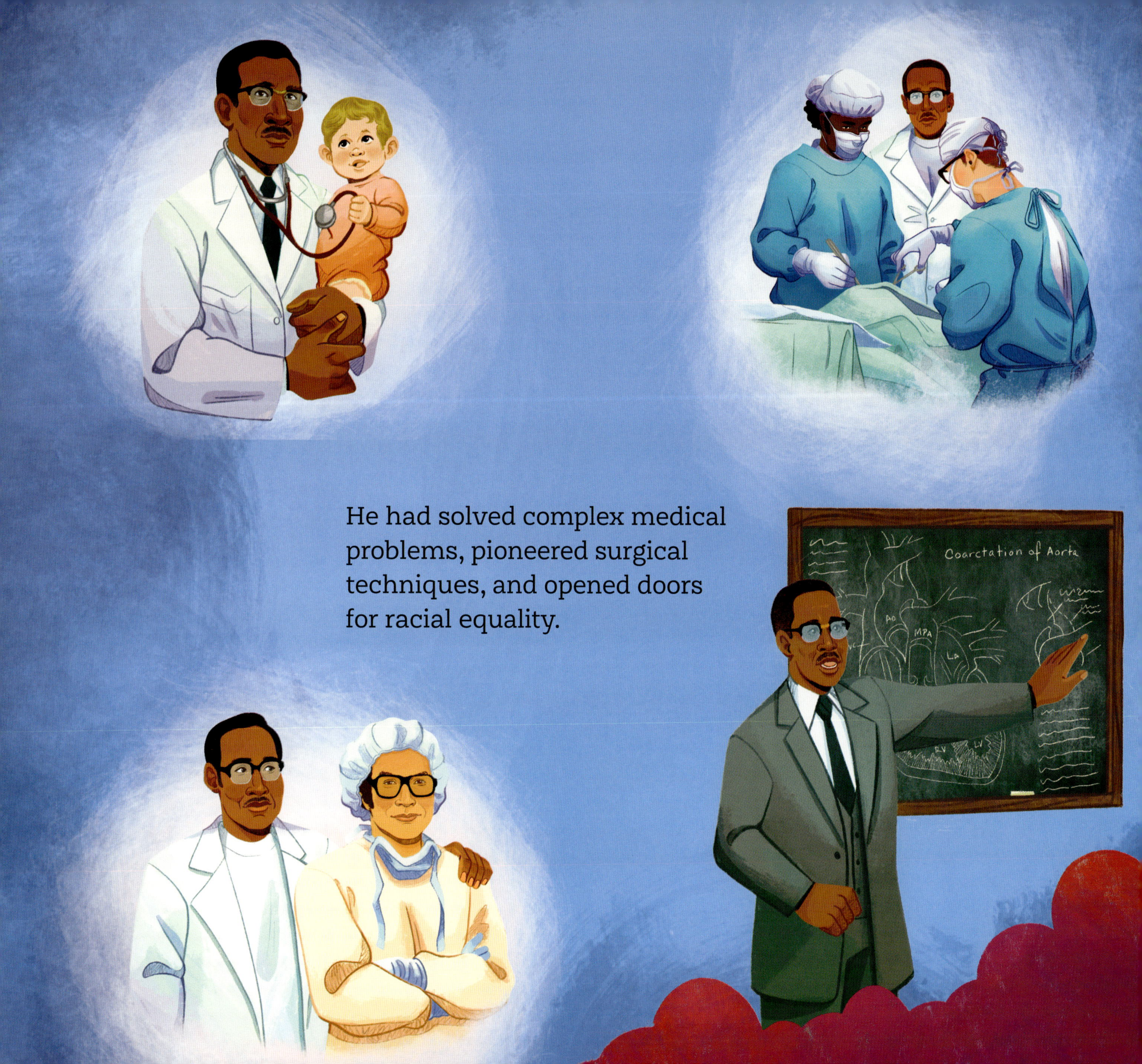

He had solved complex medical problems, pioneered surgical techniques, and opened doors for racial equality.

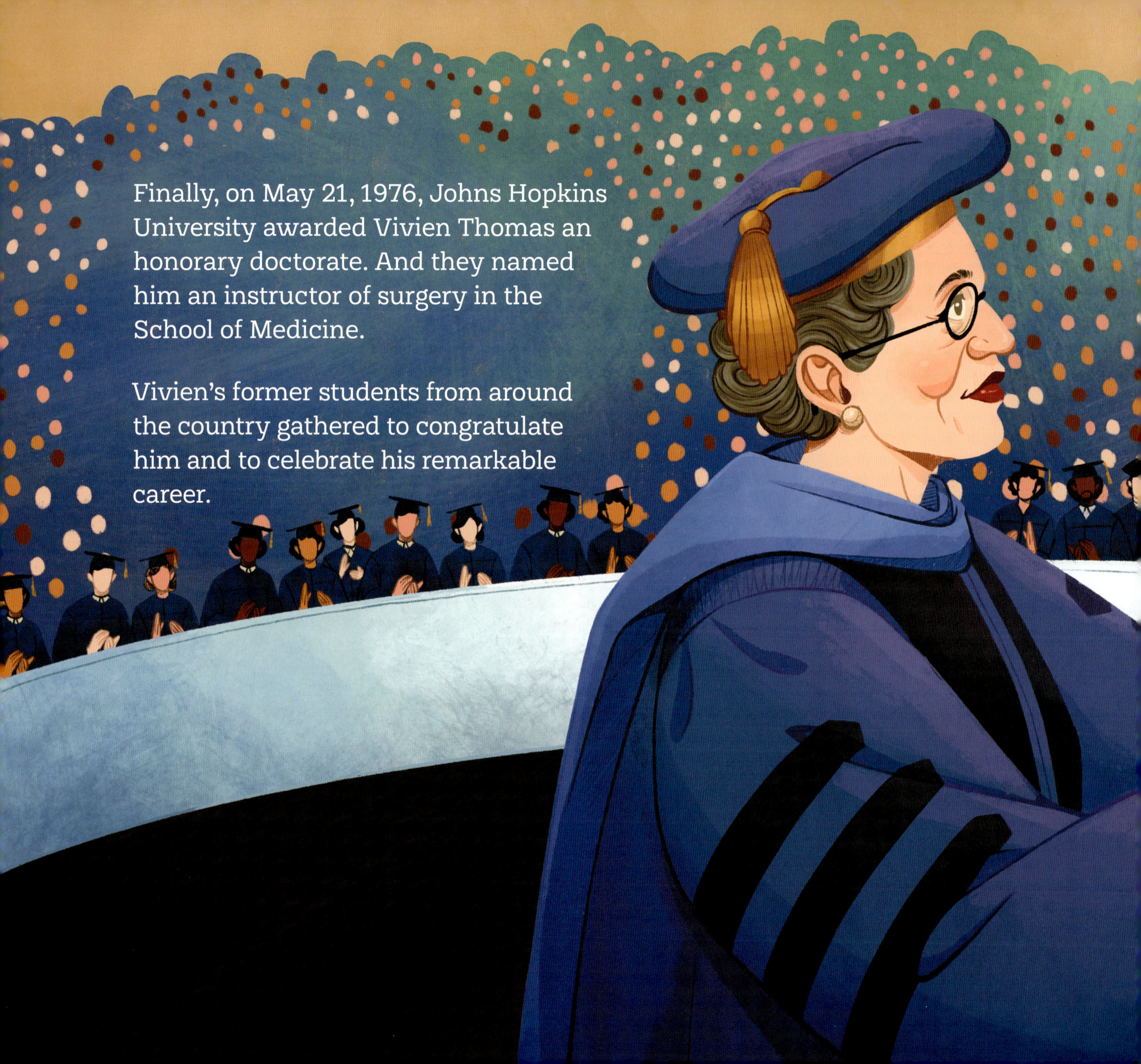

Finally, on May 21, 1976, Johns Hopkins University awarded Vivien Thomas an honorary doctorate. And they named him an instructor of surgery in the School of Medicine.

Vivien's former students from around the country gathered to congratulate him and to celebrate his remarkable career.

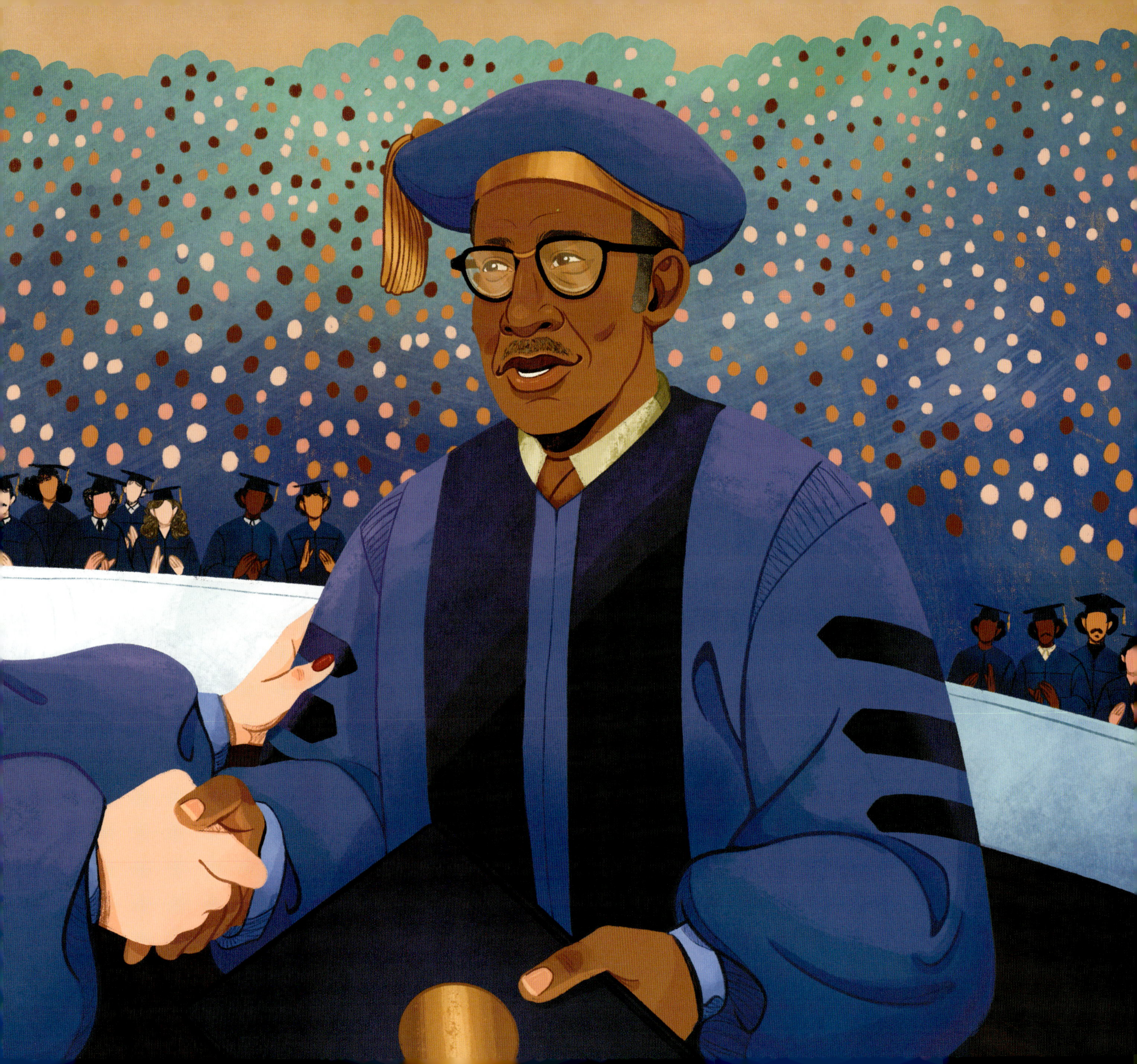

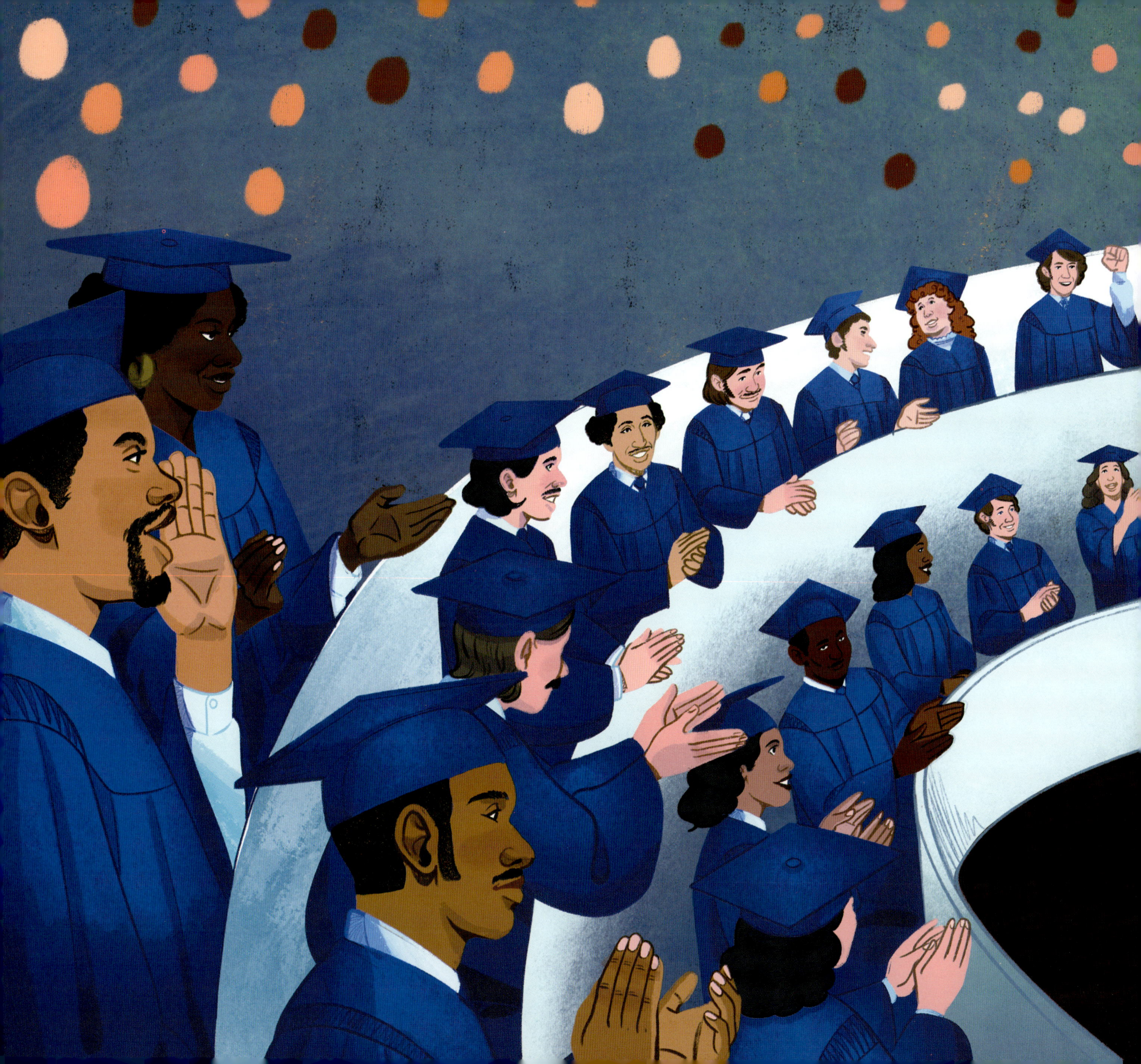

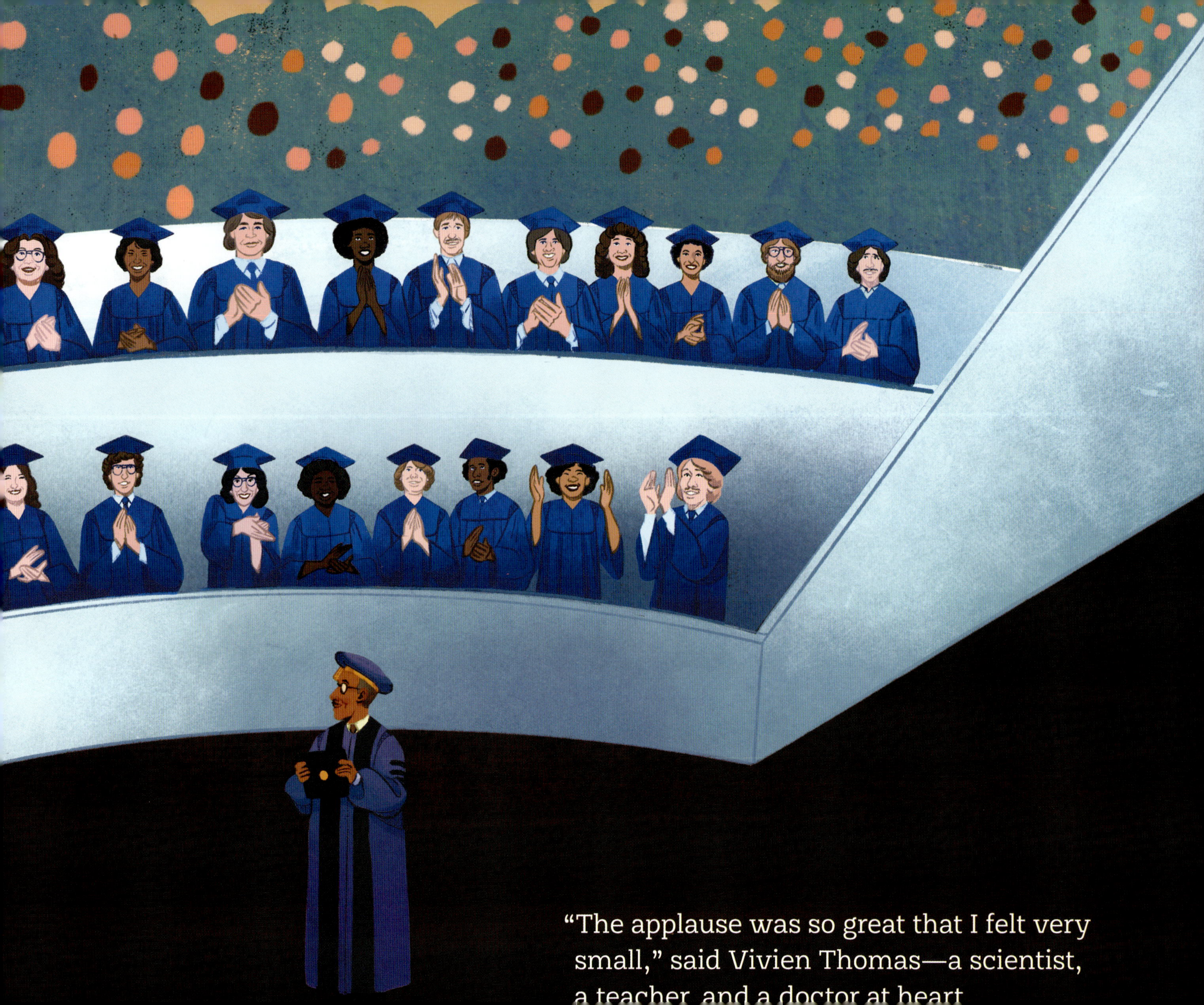

"The applause was so great that I felt very small," said Vivien Thomas—a scientist, a teacher and a doctor at heart

Author's Note

After I watched *Something the Lord Made*, a film about Vivien Thomas (1910–1985), the idea to write a picture book for young readers about this inspiring man took hold. Thomas overcame challenges, disappointments, and racial bias to become a researcher, teacher, and medical-device inventor. Along the way, he helped develop modern heart surgery.

Thomas's plan to attend college changed when his work as a carpenter slowed with a decline in the economy. Then his college savings were lost as a result of the 1929 stock market collapse. Jobs were difficult to find.

In 1930, Dr. Alfred Blalock, who was in charge of a laboratory at Vanderbilt University, hired Thomas as a laboratory assistant.

Thomas was thrilled to be working in a medical laboratory. He accepted the job at a wage lower than he earned as a carpenter, but Blalock had promised a raise. Thomas had to ask Blalock about the raise, and when Thomas looked into it, he discovered the hospital had classified and paid him as a janitor even though he performed the work of a laboratory assistant. Thomas had to ask Blalock for raises on more than one occasion. Only when Thomas threatened to leave did Blalock agree to find a way to pay him fairly.

When Blalock accepted a new job at Johns Hopkins Hospital in Baltimore, Maryland, he asked Thomas to join him. The two worked side by side in the laboratory.

But life outside the lab was different. In the hospital, racial lines were clearly drawn with segregated restrooms and a back door for Black patients. Thomas attended Blalock's parties as a bartender to earn extra money, serving drinks to men he worked with as partners during the day.

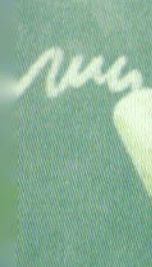

In 1944, cardiologist Helen Taussig studied infants born with blue baby syndrome. Blalock and Thomas worked with her for two years on developing a surgical procedure to cure this syndrome. It was originally called the Blalock-Taussig shunt. Not until 2023 was it renamed the Blalock-Thomas-Taussig shunt in recognition of Thomas's contributions. The surgery has helped save thousands of children born with this heart defect.

During his years of work with Blalock at Johns Hopkins Hospital, Thomas wanted to go to medical school. But he knew he would need a college degree first. He hoped colleges would give him credit for his work developing the operation to correct blue baby syndrome. But his request for credit was denied. Beginning as a freshman in college meant Thomas would be fifty years old before becoming a doctor. Sadly, he gave up on this dream.

Yet Thomas designed groundbreaking surgical equipment and devices. He helped train many surgeons on how to use the devices, which were revolutionary for heart and lung operations. A patient teacher, Thomas trained surgical residents in vascular surgery.

The surgeons Vivien trained commissioned a painting of his portrait to pay tribute to his life and accomplishments. The portrait hangs opposite Dr. Blalock's in the lobby of the Blalock Building of Johns Hopkins Hospital.

For thirty-four years, Blalock and Thomas were partners. Toward the end of Blalock's life, he said to a colleague, "I should have found a way to send Vivien to medical school."

In 1976, the faculty of the John Hopkins University School of Medicine appointed Thomas as instructor of surgery. After many years at Johns Hopkins University, Thomas received an honorary doctorate degree. Students could now call him doctor.

At home, Thomas's doctorate diploma was framed. His children's and grandchildren's graduation pictures lined the living room walls. These degrees mattered to him.

After Vivien retired, he wrote his autobiography. It was published days after he died.

Thomas's students remembered him saying, "Everybody's got a job to do. You are put here to do a job one hundred percent, regardless of how much education you have." Vivien Thomas held those words close throughout his life, and he lived them to the fullest.

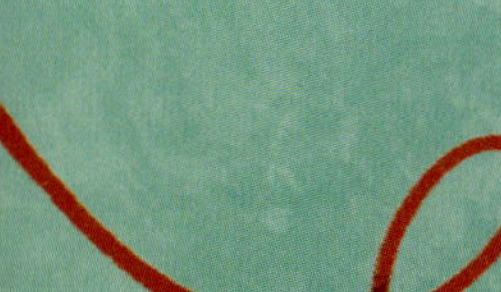

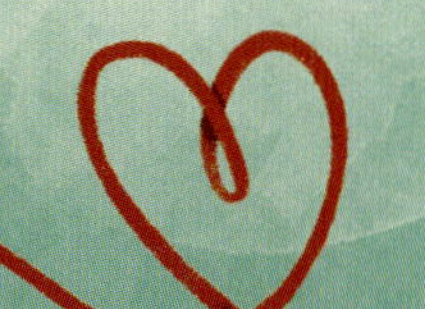

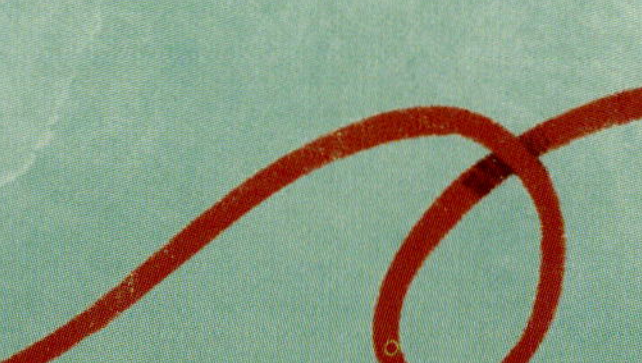

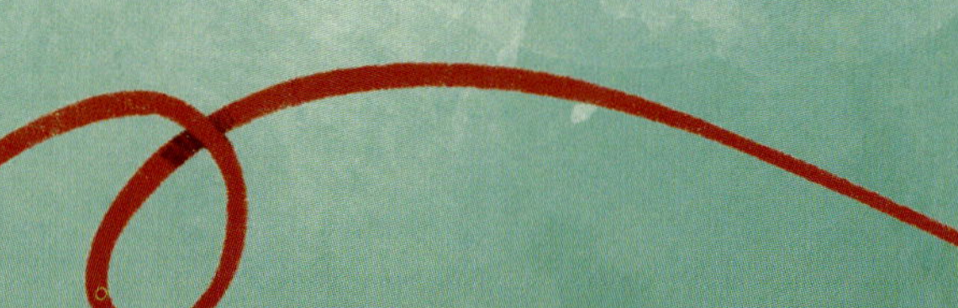

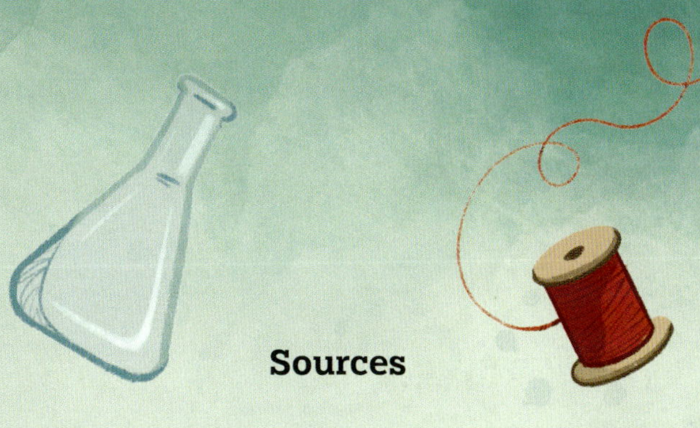

Sources

Books

Gladden, Jessie B. 2020. *A Chat with Vivien Thomas: She was the 1st to Interview Mr. Thomas on His Extraordinary Technical Discoveries Used in Dr. Alfred Blalock's "Blue Baby Operation."* iUniverse.

Pottker, Jan. 2024. *Vivien Thomas: The Man Who Overcame Racism to Save Millions of Lives*. Writer's Cramp Books.

Thomas, Vivien. 1988. *Partners of the Heart: Vivien Thomas and His Work with Alfred Blalock*. University of Pennsylvania Press.

Wyckoff, Edwin Brit. 2007. *Heart Man*. Enslow.

Video/DVD

Duke, Bill and Andrea Kalin, directors. *Partners of the Heart*, PBS documentary, 2002.

Sargent, Joseph, director. *Something the Lord Made*. HBO Films, 2004.

Internet

Hektoen International. *A Journal of Medical Humanities*. "Character, Genius, and a Missing Person in Medicine." Carrie Barron, 2019. https://hekint.org.

Washingtonian. "The Remarkable Story of Vivien Thomas, the Black Man Who Helped Invent Heart Surgery." Katie McCabe, June 19, 2020. https//www.Washingtonian.com.

Scott, H. William. *History of Surgery at Vanderbilt University*. Nashville: Vanderbilt University Medical Center, 1996.

Further Reading for Children

Hooks, Gwendolyn and Colin Bootman. 2016. *Tiny Stitches: The Life of Medical Pioneer Vivien Thomas*. Lee & Low Books.

Latta, Sara L. *Who Fixed Babies' Hearts? Vivien Thomas*. 2012. Enslow.

Williams-Newton, June and Brittany Lewis-Moore. 2024. *The Baby Heart Doctor: A Notable Black Hero who Saved Babies from "Blue Baby Syndrome."* iUniverse.

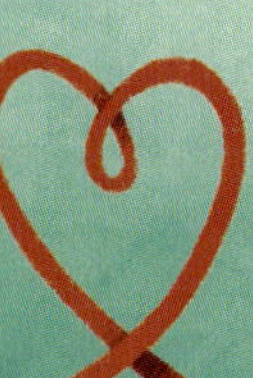

For Bob, Jason, Matt, and Nathan
—J. S.

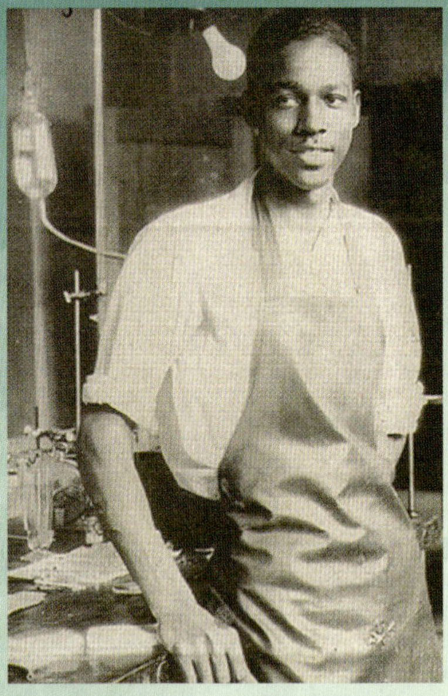
Vivien Thomas at work in the Vanderbilt University medical lab in the 1930s. Photographer unknown, public domain.

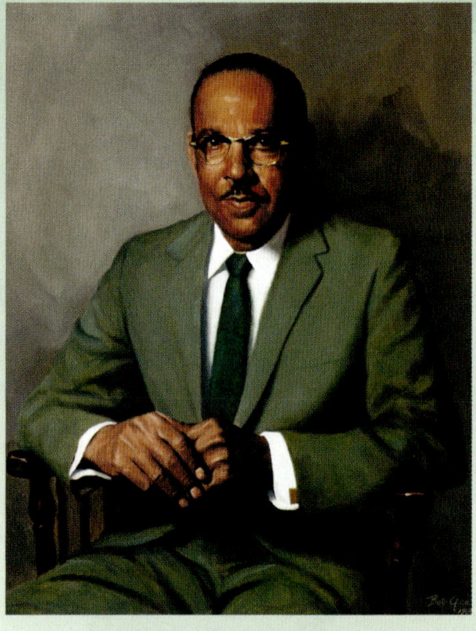
Portrait of Vivien Thomas at Johns Hopkins Hospital, mounted in 1971. Courtesy of the Chesney Medical Archives of Johns Hopkins Medical Institutions.

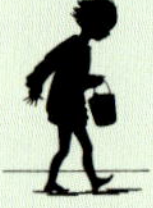

BEACH LANE BOOKS
An imprint of Simon & Schuster Children's Publishing Division
1230 Avenue of the Americas, New York, New York 10020

Book design by Greg Stadnyk

The text for this book was set in Rothwood.
The illustrations for this book were rendered in Procreate.
Manufactured in China
0126 SCP
First Edition
2 4 6 8 10 9 7 5 3 1
CIP data for this book is available from the Library of Congress.
ISBN 9781481476669
ISBN 9781481476676 (ebook)